Your Career in Healthcare

By Robert F. Wilson

President,
Wilson McLeran, Inc.
New Haven, Connecticut

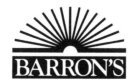

© Copyright 1996 by Barron's Educational Series, Inc.

All rights reserved.

No part of this book may be reproduced in any form, by photostat, microfilm, xerography, or any other means, or incorporated into any information retrieval system, electronic or mechanical, without the written permission of the copyright owner.

All inquiries should be addressed to:
Barron's Educational Series, Inc.
250 Wireless Boulevard
Hauppauge, New York 11788

Library of Congress Catalog Card No.: 96-1229

International Standard Book No. 0-8120-9599-5

Library of Congress Cataloging-in-Publication Data

Wilson, Robert F.
    Your career in healthcare / Robert F. Wilson.
      p. cm.
    Includes bibliographical references and index.
    ISBN 0-8120-9599-5
    1. Medicine—Vocational guidance. I. Title.
R690.W555 1996
610.69—dc20   96-1229
                                CIP

PRINTED IN THE UNITED STATES OF AMERICA
987654321

Table of Contents

Introduction vii

Acknowledgments viii

PART I   **SURVEY OF HEALTHCARE CAREERS**

Chapter 1   **Why Choose Healthcare?** 2
- Jobs for All Interests—at All Levels 3
- The Downside 5
- Making the Best Possible Healthcare Fit 6
- Another Way to Get There: *Yoga Instructor* 7
- Preparing Yourself Academically 9
- Narrowing Your Career Choices 12

Chapter 2   **Career Opportunities as Doctors** 15
Physician: M.D. and D.O. • Selected Specialties: Dermatologist, Family Physician, Gynecologist/Obstetrician, Internist, Neurologist, Otolaryngologist, Pathologist, Pediatrician, Physiatrist, Podiatrist, Proctologist, Urologist • Physician Assistant
- Another Way to Get There: *Osteopathic Doctor* 17
- Another Way to Get There: *Family Doctor* 22

Chapter 3   **Career Opportunities in Nursing** 30
Registered Nurse • Nurse Practitioner • Nurse-Midwife • Licensed Practical Nurse • Nurse Executive
- Another Way to Get There: *Certified Nurse Assistant* 39

PART II   **CAREER OPPORTUNITIES WITHIN SPECIALTIES**

Chapter 4   **Pursuing Careers in Anesthesiology** 44
Anesthesiologist • Nurse Anesthetist • Anesthesiologist Assistant
- Another Way to Get There: *Nurse Anesthetist* 48

Chapter 5   **Pursuing Careers in Cardiovascular Medicine** 51
Cardiologist • Cardiovascular Technologist • EKG Technician • Perfusionist • Respiratory Therapist

Chapter 6 **Pursuing Careers in Dentistry** **59**
Dentist • Dental Specialties: Endodontist, Oral-Maxillofacial Surgeon, Oral Pathologist, Orthodontist, Pediatric Dentist, Periodontist, Prosthodontist, Public Health Dentist • Dental Hygienist • Dental Laboratory Technician
- Another Way to Get There: *Dentist* 62
- Another Way to Get There: *Oral-Maxillofacial Surgeon*. 63

Chapter 7 **Pursuing Careers in Dietetics**. **70**
Dietitian: Business, Clinical, Community, Consultant, Educator, Management, Research • Dietetic Technician
- Another Way to Get There: *Consultant Dietitian* 72

Chapter 8 **Pursuing Careers in Eyecare** **76**
Ophthalmologist • Optometrist • Ophthalmic Medical Technician/ Technologist • Optician • Ophthalmic Laboratory Technician • Paraoptometric • Optometric Assistant • Optometric Technician

Chapter 9 **Pursuing Careers in Health Information Management** **83**
Medical Record Administrator • Medical Record Technician • Coding Specialist • Medical Transcriptionist

Chapter 10 **Pursuing Careers in Laboratory Medicine and Biomedical Engineering** **90**
Pathologist • Pathologist Assistant • Human Genetic Counselor • Technologist: Medical, Clinical Chemistry, Microbiology, Blood Bank, Immunology, Cytotechnologist • Medical Technician: Histology Technician, Phlebotomist • Biomedical Engineer
- Another Way to Get There: *Biomedical Engineer*. 97

Chapter 11 **Pursuing Careers in Mental Health** **99**
Psychiatrist • Psychiatric Technician • Psychologist • Mental Health Social Worker • Certified Alcohol and Drug Abuse Counselor • Outreach Worker • Professional Counselor
- Another Way to Get There: *Mental Health Social Worker* 105

Chapter 12 **Pursuing Careers in Speech-Language Pathology** **110**
Speech-Language Pathologist • Audiologist
- Another Way to Get There: *Speech-Language Pathologist*. 111

Chapter 13 **Pursuing Careers in Pharmacy**. **115**
Pharmacist • Pharmacist Assistant
- Another Way to Get There: *Pharmacist* 117

Chapter 14 **Pursuing Careers in Physical or Occupational Therapy**......... **120**
Physical Therapist • Physical Therapist Assistant • Occupational Therapist • Occupational Therapist Assistant
- Another Way to Get There: *Physical Therapist* 122

Chapter 15 **Pursuing Careers in Public Health** **128**
Public Health Statistician • Epidemiologist • Environmental Health Officer • Occupational Health Nurse • Health Educator
- Another Way to Get There: *Obstetrician Policy Maker*.......... 133

Chapter 16 **Pursuing Careers in Radiology**......................... **136**
Radiologist • Radiation Therapist • Radiographer • Diagnostic Medical Sonographer • Nuclear Medicine Technologist
- Another Way to Get There: *Radiologist*..................... 137

Chapter 17 **Pursuing Careers in Veterinary Medicine** **144**
Veterinarian • Veterinary Technician
- Another Way to Get There: *Research Veterinarian* 146

Chapter 18 **Jobs Available to High School Grads**.................... **150**
Animal Attendant • Dental Assistant • Dialysis Technician • Dispensing Optician Trainee • EEG Technologist Trainee • EKG Technician Trainee • Emergency Medical Technician • Home Health Aide • Medical Assistant • Nursing Aide and Psychiatric Aide
- Another Way to Get There: *Home Health Aide* 155

PART III JOB SEARCH STRATEGIES

Chapter 19 **Creating a Master Résumé and Cover Letter** **160**
- Organizing Your Résumé or C.V. 161
- Chronological and Functional Résumé Formats 162
- Targeting.. 163
- Résumé Components 164
- Formulating Your Objective and Summary 166
- Formulating Your "Experience" Section 168
- Putting Your Résumé All Together........................ 170
- Writing Your Master Cover Letter 171
- Sample Healthcare Résumés and Cover Letters.............. 173
  Physicians 177
  Nurses.. 195
  Dietitian • Optometrist • Pharmacist • Speech-Language Pathologist.. 205
  Allied Health Professionals............................ 213
  Healthcare Executives 221
  Miscellaneous Electronic Résumés...................... 231

Chapter 20 **Marketing Yourself Effectively** **256**
- Employment Agencies.................. 256
- Executive Recruiters 257
- Newspaper Want Ads and Healthcare Section Display Ads....... 258
- Trade Publication Articles and Classified Ads 260
- Database Services 260
- Industry and Function Association Officers and Members 261
- Former Coworkers and Other Professional Networks 261
- Networking Online...................... 263

Chapter 21 **Winning Interview Techniques**......................... **269**
- Know Your Prospective Employers................ 269
- Preparing for Your Interview 271
- Various Networking and Research Leads 273
- The First Interview 274
- The Second Interview 281
- Negotiating Compensation 282
- Taking Your New-Job Pulse 283

Bibliography.. **284**
- Healthcare Industry Information Sources................ 284
- Generic Job-Search Strategy and Advice.................. 286
- Scholarship, Grant, and Low-Cost Loan Sources 288

Appendix A Glossary of Basic Healthcare Terms and Abbreviations 290
Appendix B Healthcare Positions by SOC Numbers 296
Appendix C Healthcare-Related Associations......................... 298
Appendix D Career Investigation.................................. 302
- Career Investigation Checklist 302
- Information Interview with a Professional 304

Index 305

INTRODUCTION

This book was written to help job seekers in one of the following five situations:

- High school students or graduates uncertain about career direction
- College students or graduates unsure about the best way to utilize their majors
- Healthcare professionals who want to upgrade their specialty
- Healthcare professionals who want to change their specialty within the field
- Professionals outside the healthcare field who want to change careers

For readers in all of these categories, *Your Career in Healthcare* provides three kinds of essential information for a wide range of healthcare opportunities: (1) the educational and aptitudinal qualifications for entry; (2) the range of responsibilities expected; and (3) the prospects for success—both personal and financial.

Success is difficult to measure. Each of us has a different definition. In the chapters that follow, you will meet a number of people who have faced career dilemmas. Through their experiences you will see ways to get closer to your professional goal, none by itself necessarily the only way. More important, you'll learn that a false start or two at the beginning of your working life need not stifle your dreams for the healthcare career you now seek.

Most of these stories are incomplete, with the ideal job yet to be found, since careers tend to be fluid rather than static. The job that seemed perfect five years ago may hold much less appeal today. The simple truth is that these people are learning and changing as they go. You will, too.

All of the people profiled are enjoying success today at least in part because they followed solid job-search strategy. All have pursued their career goals both rigorously and systematically. *Your Career in Healthcare* passes on to you some of the strategies that worked for them. For example, it will help you:

- Determine both an interim and a long-term career path
- Prepare a marketing strategy to get you there
- Craft a master résumé and cover letters that effectively state your case for positions that interest you
- Sharpen your interviewing skills to best advance your candidacy in a variety of circumstances
- Keep a checklist on your next job to track all changes as your career goals evolve

I invite you to contact me as you work to accomplish your immediate objectives as a healthcare professional, or as you encounter problems for which I might suggest solutions. I would be pleased to consider your story for a case study in the next edition of *Your Career in Healthcare*.

R.F.W.
102676.726@compuserve.com

ACKNOWLEDGMENTS

A number of colleagues, friends, and healthcare professionals have contributed to the quality of this manuscript, among them: Martha Buchanan; David Altobelli, M.D.; Dan Austin, M.D.; Ginny Leigh-Blanchard; Larry Bouchard, MedSearch America, Inc.; George Bowersox; Janis Brown, M.D.; Nancy Cavallaro, R.D.M.S., C.N.M.; Liana Clark, M.D.; Tyler Cymet, D.O.; Marilyn Dancy, American Academy of Family Physicians; Janet Davis, S.L.P.; Fred Donini-Lenhoff, American Medical Association; Beth Faust, Health Information Management Association; Sean Gallagher; Julea Garner, M.D., American Academy of Family Physicians; David George, C.N.A.; David Greene, M.D.; James Lee Hawes, C.R.N.A.; George Hetson, D.D.S.; Pete Hines, American College of Cardiology; Jeffrey Kahn; Minna Kaufman, R.N.; Jeff Krug; Laura Kroll, American Organization of Nurse Executives; Tracy Leibach, Rensselaer Polytechnic Institute; Barry Litwin, American Medical Association; Stuart Leland, D.V.M.; Mary Linley; Al Matkowsky, C.A.D.A.C.; Pam Michael, American Dietetic Association; Lloyd Mitler, M.D.; Helaine Patterson, Yale University School of Medicine; Donna Poe, R.D.; Jocelyn Poisson, Fones School of Dental Hygiene, University of Bridgeport; Roberta Ripperger; Kenneth Rivera; Marian Rodgers; Kathleen Rooney, M.S.W.; Jennifer Sacks, American Counseling Association; Jordan Shapiro, Yale University School of Medicine; Karen Sherman; Marcia Shin; George Silvestri, U.S. Department of Labor, Bureau of Labor Statistics; Arlington Smith; Leslie Scoutt, M.D.; Joan Stenner, Yale University School of Medicine; Kim Taylor, Connecticut Hospital Association and Affiliates; Michelle Toscas, American Osteopathic Association; Mona Thomas, American Speech-Language-Hearing Association; Robert S. Tinnon; Michael Tremblay; Linda Turner, Barron's Educational Series; Bibi Vabrey; Janet Voelker, Guidance Counselor, Nashua (NH) Senior High School; Charles Williams, Principal, Conte Career Education Center New Haven, CT; Jeanne Wilson; Wooster Canine Alliance. Carol Michelini, Northwest Memorial Hospital, Chicago, made suggestions throughout the manuscript, and proposed useful ideas for additional material as well.

Consultant
Beth Guadagnoli, R.N.

Special material written by Beth Guadagnoli, Philip King, and Wendy Murphy.

Feature material on pages 6, 21, 92, 263, copyright © 1995 by the American Medical Association. Reprinted from *The Health Care Almanac*.

Résumés on pages 232, 236, 245, 246, 252, reprinted courtesy of MedSearch America, Inc., Redmond, WA.

Occupation descriptions adapted from *Occupational Outlook Handbook* (1996–1997), courtesy U.S. Department of Labor, Bureau of Labor Statistics.

PART 1
Survey of Healthcare Careers

CHAPTER 1

Why Choose Healthcare?

As a source of job opportunities these days, healthcare is hot. More than 4.3 million new health assessment, treatment, and service-related jobs will be available between 1996 and 2005, according to the U.S. Bureau of Labor Statistics—all due to growth rather than replacement. During this period, in fact, the health industry is expected to expand more than two times the rate of the economy as a whole.

Of the 30 career areas growing the fastest, 11 are in the health-services sector. The top two—personal-care aides and home-health aides—will increase by more than 100 percent between now and 2005. Other fast-growing professions include physical therapy, medical records technology, and dental hygiene. For a list of these fast-growing occupations, along with their educational requirements, see the table on page 14.

There are a number of reasons for the explosion of jobs in the healing professions. First of all, our population is getting older by the year. There are more patients and many of them are aged. Between 1990 and 2005, for example, the number of people over the age of eighty-five will grow at a rate three times that of the total population. Age groups just below this level will grow almost as fast. Much more attention is being paid to making life more livable for this growing, influential segment of the population.

Second, there is much more of an emphasis on getting healthy and staying healthy these days than was true just a generation ago. This has resulted in an increased awarenesss of the significance health has on other aspects of our lives. We now know that good health has a profound effect on the way students perform in school, for example, and how well workers do their jobs. Also (largely because our population *is* getting older), more attention is being paid to tracking the various adjustments society is making to older people, as well as to the aging process itself. Finally, our enjoyment of leisure time is closely tied to how good we feel, which in turn helps determine how healthy we are.

Key to a Healthy Old Age: Good Habits or Good Genes?

Only about 30 percent of the characteristics of aging are genetically based. The other 70 percent are not.

In other words, how most people manage old age may not be a matter of fate or genes, as many people believe. This was the conclusion of a MacArthur Foundation Consortium on Successful Aging in 1996.

The MacArthur research team, which included gerontological geneticists, psychologists, and social epidemiologists at several universities, found that staying active both physically and socially contributes to successful aging.

The team found that genetics played the greatest role in health characteristics early in life. "But by age eighty, for many characteristics there is hardly any genetic influence left," said Dr. Gerald McClearn, a research team member.

"Our basic message is that people are largely responsible for their old age," added Dr. John Rowe, team leader and director of the MacArthur Foundation.

The results were the result of a ten-year study of an often overlooked segment of the elderly population: people entering their eighties, healthy and independent. Those who continue to be productive after retirement are more likely to age successfully, the study found. "Older people should not be discouraged from doing what they think they can do," concluded Dr. Teresa Seeman, another research team member.

JOBS FOR ALL INTERESTS—AT ALL LEVELS

There has been an explosive increase in the number and variety of healthcare jobs over the past several years, with a virtual certainty of similar good news yet to come. On top of this, entirely new areas of interest and concern flourish today—preventive medicine being a striking example—creating thousands of new jobs where only a handful existed ten years ago.

A growing number of experienced medical specialists—surgeons, psychiatrists, therapists, technicians, and others—have reached career crossroads for one reason or another and are looking for alternative outlets for their expertise.

The field of public health, for example, is attracting thousands of those who have either burned out or peaked in their current careers and are looking for a greater or different challenge. As public health was conceived back in the nineteenth century, its professionals consisted largely of volunteer social workers. Technological advances and the evolution of a much more complex social fabric since then, however, have provided a structure consisting not only of physicians and nurses, but nutritionists, educators, environmentalists, planners, administrators, statisticians, and others committed to protecting the health of the public.

Public health represents an opportunity for professionals to formulate or administer policy in a familiar specialty. For example, who better than an obstetrician to determine the optimum hospital stay for birthing mothers? The reason New Jersey hospitals no longer release all new mothers the day after their babies are born is that a recently convened public health panel, including physicians for the first time, decided that for many mothers this was too short a stay, and that additional criteria for discharge should be applied. Several other states have since followed suit. (See Chapter 15 for a more comprehensive description of opportunities in the public health field.)

A New Patient Base: Computer-Users

Carpal tunnel syndrome affects two million Americans, and costs American companies $20 billion a year. With millions of schoolchildren growing up with computers and millions of correspondents abandoning the U.S. Postal Service for e-mail, that figure is expected to grow exponentially.

Carpal tunnel syndrome is a disorder of the wrist, arm, and hand caused by repetitive physical stress. Actually it has been around for more than a century, but until recently it was known to affect primarily carpenters, meat cutters, jackhammer operators, as well as pianists, baseball pitchers, and bank tellers. With the proliferation of computer use in the 1980s, though, the affliction spread to office workers, reporters, and editors.

For more information: *Relief From Carpal Tunnel Syndrome and Other Repetitive Motion Disorders*, by Nora Tannenhaus (Dell Medical Library, 1991; $3.99).

As a result of these and other sweeping changes in analagous fields, the geometrically increasing number of job opportunities make it difficult to choose among the healthcare careers. There may indeed be several kinds of jobs that would provide you with comparable levels of satisfaction and financial security, in which case the next most crucial decision is to find out which of these jobs are in sufficient demand in the marketplace. You will read more about that in the chapters to follow. On the pages ahead you will learn the educational requirements, interest areas, and personality characteristics that qualify you for openings that interest you. It will then be up to you, after meeting appropriate educational requirements, to monitor the marketplace for actual openings.

As is true in most other professions, the more education you have, the farther you are likely to go financially. But monetary reward is only one yardstick for success. Personal satisfaction is as important to some as a fat paycheck is to others. You must make up your own mind which is more important and define personal satisfaction on your own terms.

This means that an advanced degree (or for many positions even an undergraduate degree) may not be essential in attaining career satisfaction. If you have graduated from high school or completed your equivalency, there is still a wide range of possibilities for you to consider. Not only that, in many instances you will be able to go to school and still hold on to your day job (often encouraged *and sometimes paid for* by your employer), and thus be able to upgrade your skills and level in the specialty you have selected without quitting your job or taking an unpaid leave of absence. This strategy also makes it possible for you to accommodate any modified career goals that call for additional education.

THE DOWNSIDE

Unfortunately, there is another, less rosy way to look at employment potential in the healthcare industry. First of all, it is more volatile than almost any other career category in terms of job and career opportunities. Costs in every area have increased steadily over the past ten years or more, for several reasons.

The consequence of spiraling costs with the most profound potential effect on your future as a healthcare professional (this includes both newcomers and veterans) is the move toward managed care. More and more frequently, two or more healthcare providers have teamed to pool expenses and reduce costs.

This makes sense. Why should two hospitals ten blocks apart each spend $750,000 on identical computerized axial tomography equipment (a mouthful you probably will recognize as the machine providing CAT scans), when with effective scheduling a single unit could amply serve the needs of both? Multiply this example by the 27,000 hospitals nationwide as well as thousands of additional clinics of various kinds, not just for CAT scan equipment but for the myriad related capital investments they must make, and you have some idea of the financial pinch these providers face on a continuing basis.

Health maintenance organizations (HMOs) and other cost-minded insurers are affecting the bottom line in other ways. They are pressing doctors and hospitals to squeeze costs by shortening hospital stays, and in some instances switching treatments from hospitals to home care. Anesthesiologists, among the most highly paid of specialized physicians, are losing work opportunities in many instances to certified registered nurse anesthetists (CRNAs). CRNAs are licensed to perform nearly all of an anesthesiologist's functions at less than half the cost. Cost containment strikes again.

So, whether or not this country moves toward guaranteed health insurance for everyone, cost-effectiveness will remain a fact of life for everyone associated with healthcare, job seekers included. Add to this such recent phenomena as the dozens of public hospitals being sold off by some of our nation's cities, and you see an industry in the middle of a profound change.

> **Health Maintenance Organizations**
>
> Health maintenance organizations (HMOs) both finance and provide comprehensive health maintenance and treatment services to a voluntary-enrolled population for a prepaid, fixed sum. An HMO serves as both an insurer and a provider of healthcare services. In contrast to traditional health insurance, which simply reimburses covered individuals or those who provide healthcare services to them, HMOs and their providers carefully monitor and manage both the quantity and the quality of care.

Paradoxically, now and for the immediate future, the growth and creation of new jobs in some fields of healthcare is being accompanied by a loss of jobs in others. In 1994 for example, 46,000 medical school applicants competed for 16,000 places. (Harvard received 4,000 applications for a class of 165.) Also, many healthcare providers are consolidating their payrolls, which has resulted in more layoffs, individual job losses, and large-scale downsizing than the industry has ever seen. Finally, some occupations are in decline. A shortage of x-ray technicians prevalent through the 1980s no longer exists. The employment of EKG technicians similarly is expected to decrease as hospitals train registered nurses to perform basic EKG proceedures, to reduce headcount and save salary dollars.

This means that job seekers must proceed with extreme caution as they investigate and pursue specific opportunities. "Long-term potential" is a major job-search consideration, regardless of industry. You will have to keep long-term potential in mind as you prospect for employers, for at least the next decade. The two most important tools for determining the long-term potential of any opportunity are comprehensive research and skillful interviewing. Look for specific suggestions to help you master these job-search tools in Part III.

MAKING THE BEST POSSIBLE HEALTHCARE FIT

One way to better understand the healthcare industry is to consider the three means by which it mounts its assault against disease and injury: prevention, diagnosis, and treatment. Those of you drawn to one of these areas can begin to narrow your focus and begin investigations immediately. For the rest of you it will be more useful to break down the field the same way most schools do in formulating their healthcare curricula, and concentrate on one of the following three areas of study:

- Medical: Physicians and surgeons, both specialized and general practice, includes doctors of osteopathic medicine (D.O.s), whose training and education is similar to that of "allopathic" doctors of medicine (M.D.s), but who subscribe to additional holistic methodology in what is largely a preventive approach to healthcare
- Nursing: Registered and licensed practical nurses, both specialized and general practice

- Allied Health: Technologists, technicians, aides, and all other technical, support, and service occupations in various specialized areas (See Chapters 4–18, Part II.)

(Not included in either of these breakdowns are dozens of administrative, clerical, and technical occupations not specific to the healthcare field that transfer easily from industry to industry. They are virtually identical in industries such as manufacturing or food processing to their analogous positions in healthcare.)

Other significant job sources are those on the so-called fringes of healthcare, in alternative medicine (also called natural medicine). Dismissed by some medical people as ineffective, many aspects of alternative medicine are nevertheless accepted by most of the medical establishment. (Some, in fact, are part of osteopathic medicine's holistic approach.) Followers of alternative medicine emphasize diet, vitamins, and exercise for preventive care. They recommend massage, herbal remedies, and acupuncture for specific health problems. Alternative medicine is gaining momentum as a viable option because it treats people at lower cost than traditional medicine; there is less emphasis on expensive diagnostic tests and drugs. Ten states currently recognize and license naturopathic doctors, with other states reporting a thriving underground of practitioners and support people. If this is a field of interest to you, research the specific opportunities in which you might like to contribute.

ANOTHER WAY TO GET THERE

Ginny Leigh-Blanchard* holds M.A. degrees in both educational psychology and holistic health/nutrition, and has studied and practiced yoga for more than 20 years. She has taught yoga since 1982 in both the United States and Europe. Arlington Smith is a certified AIDS counselor and staff member at Affiliates for Consultation and Psychotherapy, and co-owner, with Ginny, of The Yoga Studio, in New Haven, Connecticut. Before this he was a counselor at Yale-New Haven Hospital for people with chronic and life-threatening illnesses.

GINNY: In Washington, D.C., where I was studying in 1972, there was only one holistic practitioner in the entire area. That's when I decided to finish my graduate degree in holistic health with a specialty in nutrition, which I did at Stanford University. I then started counseling anorexic and bulimic teenagers. My work with yoga began as a form of stress reduction, but it also was the best way to combine body image with nutrition and self-esteem in a way that hadn't previously been possible for me. I had the good fortune to attend the Iyengar Yoga Institute in San Francisco, and studied with some of the most senior yoga teachers in the world. I took an intensive premed curriculum, including anatomy, physiology, and kinesiology, and started substituting for other teachers.

---

*With two exceptions (noted as such), all of the 18 case study subjects profiled in *Your Career in Healthcare* chose to be identified by name, hometown, and state. Street addresses and phone numbers in the résumés they contributed, however, have been changed.

I then taught yoga on my own, both in corporations and private classes. More and more doctors are referring patients to us these days—both orthopedists and osteopathic doctors. The trend is definitely away from surgery and toward yoga, as well as other holistic alternatives. People are realizing that you can make changes on your own by stretching. You don't necessarily have to have a disc operation. The baby boomers have been assaulting themselves for years. The pounding they take from running and aerobics is incredible. Yoga also provides a safe and inexpensive way to keep joints healthy—knees being one good example. As more people recognize its benefits, they will turn to yoga—the numbers will be astounding. We're getting more and more referrals from physicians, for example, many for older women at risk for osteoporosis and who need preventive therapy. Yoga was considered a total healthcare system in India 3,500 years ago. And that's exactly what it is today.

ARLIE: In counseling AIDS patients and their families for ten years, I learned to restructure my own thinking through meditation tapes and positive thinking, among other things. Then I realized that there was a limit to how much I could transform my life just by changing my thinking. Yoga was one of the first things with a real appeal to me. That was about seven years ago, and I've been studying seriously ever since.

A lot of living in our culture is purely a cerebral experience. Yoga is a way of reversing that process to get solidly inside our bodies. There are all kinds of benefits to that. I was talking with a friend the other night whose husband was having back problems and was going to a chiropractor. I asked her if the chiropractor gave him exercises, and she said yes. I asked her if he did the exercises, and she said no.

Well, a yoga class provides motivation that a chiropractor's instructions do not. Yoga not only realigns your bones and muscles, it strengthens your body and reduces the stress on it.

The rest of this chapter will lay out many opportunities in the healthcare industry whether you are just entering the field or have been in it for some time. Those of you with experience may be burned out, plateaued, unlikely to be promoted, or for whatever other reason eager to transfer your skills and background to another specialty more suited to current interests and objectives.

PREPARING YOURSELF ACADEMICALLY

Those of you in high school or college should speak with a career or guidance counselor as soon as your interest in healthcare begins to crystallize. If your school doesn't offer career assistance, see those chapters describing your specific interest areas for the addresses of associations that can provide you with appropriate career path and educational information.

Through high schools in many city systems, students interested in one or more aspects of healthcare can complete a full course of study before they graduate. This opportunity comes as a result of local commitment and initiative, often assisted by state or federal funding. For example, at Conte Career Education Center, a magnet public high school in New Haven, Connecticut, 12 to 15 nursing aides are certified and registered every year.

"We require 120 classroom hours and 60 clinical hours," says lead teacher Minna Kaufman, who is also a registered nurse. "But with the science program the average is actually closer to 300 hours. The clinical hours consist of volunteer work at the Jewish Home for the Aged, followed by internship locally at Saint Raphael and Yale-New Haven hospitals. By the end of the program, students are familiar with nearly every duty a nursing aide will ever have." Although some Conte nursing aide students go to work immediately after graduation, most go on to college to prepare for positions requiring further education.

Conte principal Charles Williams explains: "We have an arrangement with Gateway Community-Technical College specifically geared to health careers. We designed our curriculum to mesh with theirs, in the sense that our juniors and seniors can earn up to 13 college credits if their grades are "C" or better.

"Not only that," says Williams. "Having completed the two-year program at Gateway, students have clear access to the state college and university system to pursue a four-year degree—and beyond, if they wish. We try to identify students' latent scientific interest at the middle school level, and nurture it as best we can from then on."

Though schools similar to Conte exist all across the country, such an opportunity may not be available to you. Until you get professional assistance, it probably will be best to take as many science courses as you can manage without stinting on other required courses in your core curriculum. Even if the job you want today does not require a strong science background, five years from now your situation may be completely different. Your preparation for that situation will be further along if you anticipate it now.

Most healthcare occupations require a grounding in science—particularly biology, chemistry, and physics. Let's say you find yourself in an entry-level job. The more science you have, the easier it will be for you to identify with those people around you performing more demanding tasks. The obvious consequence: Your chances for improving your work, and being promoted to a more responsible position as a result, will increase markedly. Similarly, the opportunity for you to upgrade your profession (even to doctor, if that is your interest) will be far easier to accomplish with an early exposure to science and math.

Readers interested in a career in healthcare who are coming from another field entirely should likewise read the specialty chapters ahead. Where possible, educational requirements have been delineated and information has been provided on schools offering the required courses leading to either a certificate or a degree, as indicated.

Making Career Change Happen

One way to provide focus for a career change is to fold a sheet of paper vertically, using the left-hand side to list everything you liked about your last job, and the right-hand side everything you disliked. Your objective: to find work with as many left-side points and as few right-side points as possible.

More systematic: Write your list in terms of categories, as follows:

What I Liked	What I Disliked

Position (the job itself):

. . . .
. . . .
. . . .

Function (type of work, e.g., marketing):

. . . .
. . . .
. . . .

Employer (e.g., reputation, values, location):

. . . .
. . . .
. . . .

Industry (e.g., manufacturing, financial services):

. . . .
. . . .
. . . .

Boss (direct supervisor):

. . . .
. . . .
. . . .

Using what you have written and any further thoughts you may have, complete the following work-related statements:

(At work) I need: ....
....

I am interested in: ....
....

I excel at: ....
....

I don't do well at: ....
....

I like to: ....
....

I don't like to: ....
....

I try to avoid: ....
....

I value: ....
....

Now, read over your answers and think about them.
In summary, what I've learned from this exercise about my last job is:
....
....
....

What I've learned from this exercise that may help in my next job is:
....
....
....

Changing careers obviously is a tricky business. Jumping *from* a job you do not want any more is the easy part. Jumping *to* a job that both interests you and for which you have the minimal training and educational qualifications is much tougher. The key: Look for a situation that allows you to retain as many pluses from your previous job as possible, and at the same time gives you the opportunity to discard as many negatives as caused you to leave—or consider leaving—in the first place.

To give you an idea of what educational obstacles may stand in your way for a position that interests you, consult the table on page 14, which matches the most popular healthcare occupations with the amount of education required, and indicates the growth forecast for each.

To help you decide what change might be best for you, consult the chapters just ahead.

NARROWING YOUR CAREER CHOICES

Early in this chapter we mentioned that making a specific career choice could be a very difficult decision for those of you unsure about what you want to be when you grow up. Many of today's doctors and dentists knew from an early age the kind of work they wanted to do, and from that time forward pursued their objectives both systematically and single-mindedly.

Most of the rest of us are far less driven, which makes our destination prospects considerably more murky. Either many career options seem attractive, or none does. Here's an example from somewhere between these two extremes: Let's say a position as a medical technician appeals to you. You know it includes several kinds of work that would interest you and that you could do well. Your initial reading brings you to the conclusion that there are 10 to 15 different kinds of technicians, all with similar job descriptions, responsibilities, educational requirements, and salary. You hear about laboratory technicians and cardiovascular technicians, electrocardiograph technicians and emergency medical technicians, psychiatric technicians and veterinary technicians. In addition, there are almost as many different kinds of technologists. (A technologist usually has more education and training than a technician in the same field.)

Now what? Where do you fit in? Keep an open mind; do not narrow your options until you have more data on which to base a decision. Try to learn what distinguishes each kind of technician from the rest. Does the work consist primarily of interacting with others, or would you spend a great deal of time on your own? Is there a lot of time spent manipulating data? Is it necessary to master complex equipment? What is the career path for an ambitious person?

These are all important questions, and you need the answers to them before you come to any conclusions. The information in Chapter 19 will help you put together a checklist to be sure you are pointed the right way. In Chapter 20 you will learn how to conduct an information interview to be sure the number of false starts in your new career direction is kept to a minimum. (A form to help you prepare for an information interview is provided in Appendix D.)

Meantime, unless you know exactly what kind of work you want to do next, don't minimize the importance of collecting information in helping you reach some conclusions. This book is designed to help you in this regard by providing:

- A table of contents that directs you to chapters and sections organized by job, field, and title
- Chapters that describe 14 areas of specialization
- One chapter describing ten occupations available to high school grads
- Case studies (features titled "Another Way to Get There") of 18 healthcare professionals who made career decisions their own way, for their own reasons, at a time that was right for them

- A bibliography of books and audiovisual programs on healthcare occupations, job-search advice in general, and sources for scholarships, grants, and low-cost educational loans
- A glossary of healthcare terms and abbreviations
- An appendix listing each healthcare job by the number in the *Standard Occupational Classification Manual*
- Three chapters on the job-search process, including one devoted to zeroing in on your next career option
- Dozens of résumés used by successful healthcare professionals, showing the kinds of experience and accomplishments that helped advance their careers, and how they were worded for maximum effect

Before proceeding any further in a systematic way, read through the table of contents. Keep a pencil and paper handy to jot down any career-related thoughts that occur to you, and write down page numbers when you want to return for a review of specific information.

Why Choose Healthcare?

Healthcare Jobs by Minimal Education Required†

Occupation	High School Diploma	Associate Degree (2 years)	Bachelor Degree (4 years)	Graduate Degree (5+ years)	Certification or Licensing	Growth Forecast
Ambulance Driver	*				*	A
Animal Attendant	*				*	F
Certified Coding Specialist	*				*	F
Certified Nurse Assistant	*				*	F
Dental Assistant	*					F
Dental Lab Technician	*					X
Dialysis Technician	*					F
Dispensing Optician Trainee	*					F
EEG Technologist	*					M
EKG Technician	*					D
Emergency Medical Technician	*				*	F
Licensed Practical Nurse	*				*	F
Home Health Aide	*				*	M
Medical Assistant	*				*	M
Medical Record Clerk	*					F
Nursing Aide/Psychiatric Aide	*					F
Ophthalmic Lab Technician	*					A
Optometric Assistant	*				*	A
Outreach Worker	*					F
Paraoptometric	*				*	A
Pharmacist Assistant	*					F
Accredited Record Technician		*			*	F
Cardiovascular Perfusionist		*				M
Cardiovascular Technologist		*				F
Certified Alcohol & Drug Abuse Counselor		*			*	F
Certified Medical Transcriptionist		*			*	M
Clinical Lab Technologist		*			*	A
Dental Hygienist		*			*	M
Medical Sonographer		*			*	F
Nuclear Medicine Technologist		*			*	M
Occupational Therapist Assistant		*			*	M
Ophthalmic Medical Techologist		*				A
Optician		*			*	F
Pharmacy Technician		*				A
Physical Therapist Assistant		*				M
Psychiatric Technician		*				F
Radiographer		*				F
Respiratory Therapist		*			*	M
Registered Nurse		*			*	F
Veterinary Technician		*				F
Dietitian			*		*	F
Medical Record Administrator			*		*	M
Medical Social Worker			*			F
Occupational Therapist			*		*	M
Pharmacist			*		*	F
Physical Therapist			*		*	M
Physician Assistant			*		*	F
Radiation Therapist			*		*	M
Anesthesiologist Assistant				*	*	M
Audiologist				*	*	F
Genetic Counselor				*	*	F
Nurse Anesthetist				*	*	M
Nurse Executive				*	*	F
Nurse Midwife				*	*	F
Nurse Practitioner				*	*	M
Pathologist Assistant				*	*	M
Speech-Language Pathologist				*	*	M
Optometrist				*	*	A
Dentist				*	*	A
Physician				*	*	F
Professional Counselor				*	*	F
Veterinarian				*	*	A

†With additional formal or on-the-job training.

GROWTH FORECAST
A - As fast as average
X - Static
F - Faster than average
D - Declining
M - Much faster than average

CHAPTER 2
Career Opportunities as Doctors

One way to decide which area of healthcare you want to work in is to find out how much time and talent you need to get there. Part II of *Your Career in Healthcare* covers this information in 14 different specialty areas, including details about the responsibilities and rewards of these positions.

This information is intended to make you aware of the tools you'll need to reach the professional goal that most interests you, or at least to help you narrow your focus.

"Doctor" is the first word that comes to mind when anyone mentions the words "career in healthcare." In this chapter, you will read about opportunities as doctors as well as several specialized careers stemming from the profession. (Ten healthcare occupations that require no more than a high school diploma are described in Chapter 18 at the end of Part II.)

All of the professions dealt with in this book are discussed in terms of five criteria:

1) *Personality traits and skills most likely to facilitate success*
2) *Academic preparation required or desired*
3) *Typical duties*
4) *General job outlook*
5) *Average potential earnings*

In this chapter you'll find out what it takes to become a doctor, as well as the responsibilities and rewards in store for those who qualify. A number of physician specialties not covered in Part II are described, along with the names and addresses of professional associations that can provide specific information about them. Chapter 3 focuses similarly on the nursing profession.

PHYSICIAN

M.D. and D.O.

Medical doctors (M.D.s) and osteopathic doctors (D.O.s) require more education and work longer hours than probably any other category of healthcare professional. They are also the most highly paid. Beyond these generalizations, several other factors should be considered.

PREREQUISITES

Men and women who want to be doctors must have a desire to serve patients, be self-motivated, and be able to survive both day-to-day pressures and long hours of study. Medical *residents* (graduate students) are on call 24 hours a day during work weeks of 80 hours or more.

Physicians also must be willing to study throughout their career to keep up with medical advances. They should have a good bedside manner, emotional stability, and the ability to make the right decisions in emergencies.

What Makes a Good Doctor?

When medical student Asif Kidwai used an Internet forum to ask doctors what traits distinguish excellent physicians from mediocre ones, he was gratified by the response. Over a period of several weeks Kidwai compiled these replies to his query, and included them as part of a return message of thanks. Here is the "List of Desirable Qualities in a Physician," as received from the doctors who participated:

- Unquestionable integrity; highly principled
- Forthright
- Naturally energetic and enthusiastic
- Genuinely concerned about the problems of others
- Orderly, logical mind; mentally efficient
- Understanding
- Motivated by idealism, compassion, and service
- Confidence-inspiring
- Calm in critical and stormy situations
- Able and willing to learn from others
- Conscientious
- Wise, thoughtful, able to get to the heart of a problem
- Observant
- Adaptable, able to adjust to new knowledge and changing conditions
- Considerate, courteous, and tactful

PREPARATION

The minimum educational requirement for entry to one of the nation's 141 medical schools—including 18 schools teaching osteopathic medicine—is three years of college. Most applicants, however, have at least a bachelor's degree. Required premedical study includes undergraduate work in physics, biology, and chemistry, in addition to the college courses everybody else takes: English, mathematics, and the social sciences among them.

Acceptance to medical school is extremely competitive. Applicants must submit transcripts, scores from the Medical College Admission Test (MCAT), and letters of recommendation. Character, personality, leadership qualities, and participation in extracurricular activities are other factors considered.

Medical school usually takes four years. The first two are spent primarily in laboratories and classrooms taking such courses as anatomy, biochemistry, pathology, pharmacology, microbiology, medical ethics, and medical law. Students learn to examine patients, recognize symptoms, and take medical histories. The last two years students work as *interns,* learning to diagnose and treat patient illnesses under the supervision of experienced physicians. They also take on rotating assignments in internal medicine, family practice, obstetrics and gynecology, pediatrics, psychiatry, and surgery, and other areas of specialty.

Based on their experiences in these rotating assignments, as well as other information, students begin the arduous process of selecting the specialty within which they will work on a full-time basis as doctors.

After medical school comes residency, the graduate school of medical education. To qualify, each candidate for M.D. or D.O. must pass an examination by the National Board of Medical Examiners. Those who want to specialize can take as long as seven more years in residency. (See the table on page 20 for a list of M.D.s by specialty.) If they seek board certification by the American Board of Medical Specialists, M.D.s must pass yet another exam after residency, in some cases after one or two years of practice. All states require physicians to successfully complete a state licensing examination before they can legally practice. Although doctors licensed in one state can usually get a license to practice in another without further examination, some states require individual licensure. Graduates of most foreign medical schools can generally begin practice in the United States after passing an exam and completing a hospital residency training program.

ANOTHER WAY TO GET THERE

Tyler C. Cymet, D.O., graduated in 1988 from Nova Southeastern University College of Osteopathic Medicine in Florida. He completed his residency in internal medicine at Yale University School of Medicine, with an additional year as chief medical resident at Sinai Hospital of Baltimore. In the following paragraphs, Dr. Cymet traces his choice of osteopathic medicine as a career, his subsequent concentration on primary care, and some of the distinctions between allopathic (M.D.) physicians and osteopathic (D.O.) physicians:

As people develop, they decide what to do with their lives. Those who choose medicine have further decisions to face: Do they want to work with people? Do they want to work with data? Do they want the responsibility of being a doctor, or would they prefer a technician or laboratory role?

Those who decide to be doctors have more decisions. Do they want to specialize and treat one specific part of the body, or do they want to take care of the whole person—treating not only physical needs but social and psychological needs as well? Being an osteopathic physician means treating the whole person, and for those with this philosophy the best training is in osteopathic medical school.

I came to this conclusion largely because of family. Cousins of mine who are chiropractors taught me about manipulation and its role in healthcare. Unfortunately, chiropractors are specialists without generalist training. They specialize in musculoskeletal disease, but they don't know as much as they need to about the people they care for.

Osteopathic medicine gave me the broadest range of possibilities. My philosophy of medicine was that of an osteopathic physician. No matter what I did I wanted to spend time with people, and I believed that taking care of the whole person was important.

After my third year of college I went to Northwestern School of Medicine for a semester. The philosophy there was, whatever you do, be the best at it. This was fine, but while I was there they were training only specialists. I could have continued in the six-year medical program and become an M.D. (or gone to Chicago Medical School, which also accepted me), but I realized that training as an osteopathic doctor was the best route to treating the whole person. In most allopathic schools, you can start doing radiology your first day as an intern, and never deliver a baby. In rotation as an osteopathic intern you not only deliver babies, you take all of the responsibility a doctor takes in *making the decision* to deliver a baby.

Here's another distinction: An osteopathic physician says "What is the cause of the problem?" not "What is the problem?" So if a patient comes in with swollen legs, you don't say: "How do I get the swelling down?" You say: "Why are the legs swollen?"

I realize D.O.s are a minority profession, compared to M.D.s. Minorities are looked at differently, and often have to explain themselves. We're not going to outgrow M.D.s—not when there are 600,000 of them and 38,000 of us. But that's all right. I get a tremendous amount of respect from my patients, and I love the position I have in this community as a physician.

> If people look at me and another doctor and say he's a better doctor because he's an M.D., what can I do about it? I'm practicing medicine with the philosophy I believe in, and doing what I think is best for my patients. And that makes me feel good about myself.

PRINCIPAL DUTIES

Both medical doctors and doctors of osteopathic medicine treat disease and injury, but D.O.s consider all body systems as interrelated and dependent upon one another for good health. They put particular emphasis on the musculoskeletal system: bones, muscles, ligaments, and nerves. In addition to all of the medication and surgical remedies used by M.D.s, D.O.s offer osteopathic manipulative treatment as well for some kinds of back pain, neck pain, headaches, and other medical conditions.

Approximately 61 percent of all D.O.s and 34 percent of all M.D.s are primary care physicians who, unlike specialists, see the same patients on a regular basis for a variety of ailments and preventive treatments. Primary care physicians consist of pediatricians, general and family doctors, and internists. Most family doctors provide obstetric care, as well. When appropriate, primary care physicians refer patients to other specialists including neurologists, radiologists, orthopedists, and dermatologists.

Return of the Family Doc

The primary care movement has almost single-handedly brought back the general practitioner (G.P.). Before World War II, most doctors were G.P.s, also known as family doctors. Dealing with heart problems as readily as broken bones, they delivered babies and treated terminal cancer patients with equal facility.

But World War II and the Korean War changed the medical profession profoundly, most dramatically of all in emergency medicine. The staggering number and variety of battlefield injuries forced doctors to exercise unprecedented creativity. The resulting innovations and inventions inevitably found their way home, leading to civilian applications that forever changed the way medicine is practiced. Two of the major antibiotics used to save lives today, streptomycin and para-amino salicyclic acid, were discovered in 1943.

(The following tables list the top ten M.D. and D.O. specialties by percentage.)

Top Ten M.D. Specialties by Percentage

1. Internal Medicine	16.5
2. General and Family Practice	10.7
3. Pediatrics	6.9
4. General Surgery	5.7
5. Psychiatry	5.5
6. Obstetrics and Gynecology	5.3
7. Anesthesiology	4.4
8. Orthopedic Surgery	3.1
9. Diagnostic Radiology	2.8
10. Cardiovascular Diseases	2.6
	63.5
Other specialties	23.1
Unspecified/unknown	13.4
Total	100.0%

Source: American Medical Association, 1993

Top Ten D.O. Specialties by Percentage

1. Family Practice	46.6
2. Internal Medicine	7.3
3. Emergency Medicine	6.3
4. Anesthesiology	4.2
5. Psychiatry	2.5
6. General Surgery	2.5
7. Orthopedic Surgery	2.4
8. Pediatrics	2.4
9. Obstetrics and Gynecology	2.2
10. Cardiology	1.5
	77.9
Other specialties	19.2
Unknown/unspecified	2.9
Total	100.0%

Source: American Osteopathic Association, 1995

SELECTED SPECIALTIES

Most physicians prefer private practice. Others teach in medical schools or teaching hospitals, work only in research, or are salaried employees of hospitals, health maintenance organizations, or other prepaid healthcare plans. A number of specialties are treated in separate chapters in Part II. Others are described briefly below. Names and addresses of professional associations that can provide specific program and career path information follow each entry. (A more complete list of generic associations can be found in Appendix C.)

A Smattering of Specialists

In the August 24–31, 1994 issue of the *Journal of the American Medical Association,* Dr. Spence Meighan reported his failure to come up with a collective noun appropriate for all doctors. "We are so specialized," he wrote, "that no single collective noun can represent the rich diversity of talent that graces our distinguished profession." His mock solution was to match selected specialties with his own collective nouns. Here is a partial list:

- A *block* of anesthesiologists
- A *murmur* of cardiologists
- A *rash* of dermatologists
- A *pool* of geneticists
- A *wrinkle* of geriatricians
- A *smear* of gynecologists
- A *drill* of neurosurgeons
- A *nest* of obstetricians
- A *scrimmage* of sports medicine physicians
- A *puddle* of urologists

Dermatologist

Dermatologists treat diseases and problems of the human skin, hair, and nails. Their patients may be troubled with something as common as warts or acne, or as serious as cancer. Dermatologists treat boils, abscesses, skin injuries, or infections. They remove lesions, cysts, birthmarks, and other growths. They also treat scars and perform hair transplants.

    Resource: **American Academy of Dermatology**
                          930 N. Meacham Road
                          Schaumburg, IL 60168

Family Physician

Family physicians are concerned with the total healthcare of the individual and the family. They perform surgery, care for the seriously ill in hospital critical care units, handle major trauma cases, staff a hospital, and deliver babies, including performing cesarean sections. Many family physicians develop an area of special expertise, such as sports medicine, geriatrics, preventive care, women's health, adolescent health, or research.

Resource: American Academy of Family Physicians
8880 Ward Parkway
Kansas City, MO 64114

ANOTHER WAY TO GET THERE

In 1981, at age thirty-three, Dan Austin was a building and electrical contractor in northern Idaho. His wife, Sandy, a teacher, was about to give birth to their first child. For a number of months Dan had shared with Sandy a vague sense of dissatisfaction—that perhaps he could be doing more for humanity than building houses.

"I was thinking family physician," says Dan now. "I knew I had the intellectual capacity, but I had no idea what doors would be open or shut, or how I'd respond to being back in school as a new dad—not to mention all the financial hardships."

After finishing high school in 1966, Dan had a half-formed idea of joining the ministry, and enrolled at the University of California at Santa Barbara. "I was a kid who grew up with some compassion and basic intelligence, but no real direction," he recalls. He earned a degree in math, but didn't quite see how it fit into the real world.

So instead of worrying about a career he took off for the back country, backpacking and mountaineering in the Sierras, Mexico, Argentina, and Alaska—including a climb up Mount McKinley. He dabbled in grad school, worked part-time, and taught math in a middle school. Then he fell in love, got married, and dove into his teaching career fulltime.

Five years later, still feeling the pull of the western wilderness, he and Sandy quit their teaching jobs, sold the house and moved to Sand Point, Idaho. She found a new teaching job; he started a construction business, building and rehabilitating and moving houses. Neither of them was making much money, but they didn't care. They were too busy enjoying life.

Then came Dan's doubts about what he was doing with his life. They decided that he would go back to school. Encouraged by the family doctor who had delivered his daughter, Dan signed up at Whitworth College, 75 miles west in Spokane, as a fifth-year grad student without a degree objective. What he really wanted to do, though, was meet premed requirements.

"It was unbelievable. Here I was, thirty-four and a brand-new dad, and the first course I took was developmental biology and embryo development. I went nuts; I had never had such a love of education in my life. I didn't care about grades—I just loved what I was learning."

Finishing the premed courses took two years; nights and summers Dan taught math classes that included some of the same kids who were his classmates during the day. A few medical schools he applied to thought this middle-aged guy must be purely on a lark, but once the admissions people interviewed him they realized how serious he was. Of the several schools at which he was accepted, Dan chose Dartmouth Medical School.

Now including a six-week-old baby boy, the family packed up and headed for northern New England. The first two years, Dan's grades fell off a little as his priorities broadened to include quality time with his family and tutoring a few classmates. He recalls skipping a complete lecture on birthing one afternoon to pick up his daughter at day care. Yet he finished med school in the top 15 percent of his class.

Sandy taught while Dan studied. He was helped with tuition by federal health education loans, as well as the Dartmouth scholarship fund. The scholarship was one of the benefits of being an older-than-usual student—it was based on the income of students' parents, who in Dan's case were by this time retired. Still, he ended up about $60,000 in debt.

Dan was open-minded about specialty—even while doing his third-year obstetrics rotation at Martin Luther King Hospital in Los Angeles. During one three-week stretch at the hospital Dan figures he delivered more than 50 babies. The obstetrics rotation was followed by rotations in psychiatry, internal medicine, pediatrics, and surgery, all of which he enjoyed. He discovered that he liked family practice best of all, which gave him the opportunity to work in several specialties.

Dan's first day as a practicing family doctor was September 3, 1991, his daughter's tenth birthday, and ten years to the day since the decision to leave Idaho. Today he has a practice of 2,500 patients in Bellingham, Washington, with five other doctors.

Dan is deeply involved in medical politics and medical organizations. He has served on multiple committees of the Washington and American Academies of Family Physicians, and chairs the state chapter's legislative commission. "I was also the only male member of the American Academy Women's Committee. Any way I can, I want to improve universal patient access to healthcare."

Sandy is assistant principal at a local middle school, and works just as hard as Dan does. A lot has changed for them in the past 15 years, but they're still enjoying life.

"I'm a guy who loves to do it all," Dr. Austin says. "I look back and wonder why it took me so long. But once I figured it out, I was never more sure about anything. I see some guys who are only thirty and burned out. I just turned forty-eight and *feel* thirty.

Gynecologist/Obstetrician

Gynecologists and obstetricians are concerned with the health of a woman's reproductive system. Gynecologists specialize in treating diseases and disorders of nonpregnant women; obstetricians provide medical care before, during, and after childbirth. Some physicians handle both specialties.

> Resource: American College of Obstetricians/Gynecologists
> 409 12th Street, NW, #300
> Washington, DC 20024

Internist

Internists diagnose and treat diseases and injuries of human internal organ systems. They employ diagnostic images and tests, using medical instruments and equipment. They prescribe medication and recommend dietary and activity programs, as diagnosed.

> Resource: American Society of Internal Medicine
> 2011 Pennsylvania Avenue NW, Suite 800
> Washington, DC 20006

Neurologist

Neurologists, often called brain specialists, diagnose and treat functional or organic disorders of the nervous system, which includes the brain, spinal cord, and nerves. Neurologists use an electroencephalograph (EEG) to measure brain waves and thus diagnose and evaluate head trauma, strokes, infectious diseases, epilepsy, brain tumors, and other problems.

> Resource: American Board of Neurological Surgery
> 6550 Fannin Street, Suite 2139
> Houston, TX 77030

Otolaryngologist

Otolaryngologists are ear, nose, and throat specialists. They treat patients with hearing loss or speech loss from disease or injury, prescribe medications, and may perform surgery. A physician may decide to specialize in only one type of disorder: ear (otologist), nose (rhinologist), or throat (laryngologist).

> Resource: American Board of Otolaryngology
> 5615 Kirby Drive, Suite 936
> Houston, TX 77005

Pathologist

Pathologists study the nature, cause, progression, and effects of diseases. They perform tests on body tissues, fluids, secretions, and other specimens to see if a disease is present and to determine its stage. They perform autopsies to find out why a person died and to study the effects of medical treatment. Pathologists often specialize in areas such as clinical chemistry, microbiology, or blood banking. They may supervise the pathology department of a medical school, hospital, clinic, medical examiner's office, or research institution. (See also Chapter 10, Pursuing Careers in Laboratory Medicine and Biomedical Engineering.)

Resources: American Society of Clinical Pathologists
2100 W. Harrison Street
Chicago, IL 60612

U.S. and Canadian Academy of Pathology
3643 Walton Way
Augusta, GA 30909

Pediatrician

Pediatricians specialize in the development and care of children, and the diagnosis and treatment of childhood diseases. They are concerned with behavioral and social problems, as well as specific medical aspects of child health.

Resource: American Academy of Pediatrics
141 N.W. Point Boulevard
Elk Grove Village, IL 60007

Physiatrist

Physiatrists specialize in the use of physical devices and exercise to rehabilitate patients. They determine the kind of therapy needed; prescribe exercises or treatments using light, heat, cold, or other processes; and instruct the physical therapists who administer these treatments. They also recommend occupational therapy for patients who must remain hospitalized for long periods of time or for those who must change their work because of a disability.

Resource: Association of Academic Physiatrists
5987 E. 71st Street
Indianapolis, IN 46220

Podiatrist

Podiatrists, also known as doctors of podiatric medicine, diagnose and treat disorders, diseases, and injuries of the foot and lower leg. They treat corns, calluses, ingrown toenails, bunions, heel spurs, and arch problems; ankle and foot injuries, deformities, and infections; and foot complaints associated with diseases such as diabetes. They prescribe drugs, order physical therapy, set fractures, and perform surgery. Podiatrists also fit corrective inserts called orthotics, design plaster casts to correct deformities, and design custom-made shoes.

Resource: American Association of Colleges of Podiatric Medicine
1350 Piccard Drive, Suite 322
Rockville, MD 20850

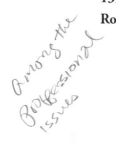

Proctologist

Proctologists treat diseases and disorders of the anus, rectum, and colon. They may prescribe medication and recommend changes in the patient's living habits or may perform surgery to remove or repair the affected organ or tissues.

>   Resource: **American Society of Colon and Rectal Surgeons**
>   **85 W. Algonquin Road, Suite 550**
>   **Arlington Heights, IL 60005**

Urologist

Urologists treat disorders of the urinary system of both men and women, and of the reproductive organs of men. They may prescribe medicines for simple ailments, such as a bladder infection, or perform surgery for more complicated conditions, such as kidney stones or an enlarged prostate gland.

>   Resource: **American Urological Association**
>   **1120 N. Charles Street**
>   **Baltimore, MD 21201**

OUTLOOK

In 1992, approximately half a million physicians were at work in this country, two thirds of them in office-based settings such as clinics and HMOs. From 1996 through the year 2005, employment of physicians is expected to grow faster than the average for all occupations. As you may remember from Chapter 1, the healthcare industry is expanding, both because more people are becoming aware of getting healthy and staying healthy, and because our aging population requires increased medical attention.

Job prospects are best for primary care physicians and for geriatric and preventive care specialists. In general, job prospects nationwide are worst in the Northeast and the West, where the ratio of physicians to the general population in urban areas is highest, and best in the South and Southwest, where the ratio of physicians to general population is much lower. A shortage of doctors also exists in many rural and low-income regions throughout the country. Some M.D.s and D.O.s find these areas unattractive because of low earning potential and isolation from medical colleagues; many also prefer the faster pace of an urban environment. Others, however, find the rewards and challenges of working with the medically underserved both personally and professionally fulfilling.

Many new physicians avoid solo practice and take salaried jobs in group medical practices, clinics, and HMOs because of the regular hours and the opportunity to consult with peers. Others go for salaried positions because they can't afford the high medical malpractice insurance or the cost of setting up a private practice while they pay off their student loans.

EARNINGS

According to the American Medical Association, the median net income (after expenses) for all U.S. physicians was $189,300 in 1994. Self-employed physicians—owners or part-owners of their practices—averaged somewhat more than did doctors who worked for others. Earnings also varied according to specialty, number of years in practice, geographic region, hours worked, skill, personality, and professional reputation. (The following table lists physician annual earnings by specialty.)

Top Ten M.D. Categories by Salary*

1. Surgery	$262,700
2. Radiology	$259,800
3. Anesthesiology	$224,100
4. Obstetrics/Gynecology	$221,900
5. Pathology	$197,300
6. Internal Medicine	$180,800
7. Pediatrics	$135,400
8. Emergency Medicine	$135,000
9. Psychiatry	$131,300
10. General/Family Practice	$116,800
All physicians	$189,300

* Mean net income after expenses

Source: AMA Socioeconomic Monitoring System, 1994

PHYSICIAN ASSISTANT

Being a physician assistant (PA) is a great career choice for people who are unable or unwilling to make the commitment in time, expense, or scholarship to become a physician. Physician assistants practice medicine under the supervision of licensed D.O.s or M.D.s, providing various health services that until a few years ago were the province of the physician. In 1970, there were fewer than 100 PAs; today there are about 25,000.

PREREQUISITES

Physician assistants come into direct contact with patients on a continuing basis, often as the initial patient contact, and therefore deal with all kinds of people. For this reason they must be mature, emotionally stable, empathic, and decisive. Like physicians, PAs spend much of their day standing or walking.

PREPARATION

To qualify for physician assistant training, many programs require applicants to have completed at least two years of college in the arts and sciences and to have had some work experience in healthcare. Most PA programs last two years, and are conducted in medical schools, community colleges, schools of allied health, or hospitals. Included are courses in biochemistry, nutrition, human anatomy, physiology, microbiology, clinical pharmacology, clinical medicine, geriatric and home healthcare, disease prevention, and medical ethics. Course study is followed by rotated, hands-on study in specialties such as family medicine, general surgery, emergency medicine, obstetrics and gynecology, and ambulatory psychiatry. Rotations are often supervised by physicians who want to hire a PA, and can lead to permanent employment.

As of 1996, 46 states require physician assistants to pass a certifying exam open only to graduates of accredited educational programs. To remain certified, PAs must have 100 hours of continuing medical education every two years and pass a recertification examination every six years.

PRINCIPAL DUTIES

Physician assistants always work under the supervision of a physician. Many PAs, however, work in rural or inner-city clinics, where a physician is available perhaps only one or two days a week. In these situations, PAs provide most of the patients' healthcare, and otherwise consult with the supervising physician by phone. Other PAs may make house calls, or check on hospitalized patients and report back to the physician. The duties of PAs who specialize vary widely with the demands of the specialty. Almost half of all practicing physician assistants are in primary care. Family practice is the most common specialty for physician assistants (33 percent), followed by surgery and surgical subspecialties, general internal medicine, and emergency medicine.

OUTLOOK

Employment opportunities are projected as excellent for physician assistants. The number of men and women working as PAs is expected to grow faster than the average for all occupations through the year 2005, partially to provide primary care and enable physicians to spend a larger percentage of their time on more complicated tasks.

EARNINGS

The average salary for all PAs in 1995, according to the American Academy of Physician Assistants, was between $55,000 and $60,000, although the upper range can exceed $100,000. Salaries vary by specialty, geographical location, and experience.

Resources: American Academy of Physician Assistants
950 North Washington Street
Alexandria, VA 22314

Executive Director
Accreditation Review Committee on Education
   for the Physician Assistant
1000 N. Oak Avenue
Marshfield, WI 54449

See Chapters 4–18 for names and addresses of organizations providing further information about physician licensure and accreditation, residency application, and education in medical specialties. For information on scholarships, grants, and low-cost loan sources for medical students, see the Bibliography.

CHAPTER 3
Career Opportunities in Nursing

Nurses complement the job of the physician by focusing on patient *response* to actual or potential health problems. Nurses are educated to be attuned to the whole person, not just specific illnesses or injuries. While a medical diagnosis may be fairly defined, the human response to a health problem may be much more fluid and variable, and may have a significant impact on a person's ability to overcome the initial medical problem. According to the American Nurses Association, "It is often said that physicians *cure* and nurses *care*." Or, in the words of Florence Nightingale, nursing is "having charge of the personal health of somebody . . . and to put that patient in the best condition for nature to act upon him."

Nurses' broad-based education and holistic focus positions them as the logical centerpiece on which to build the healthcare system of the future. People are coming to realize that they must take increased responsibility for their own health. The professionals most likely to help make this happen are nurses.

REGISTERED NURSE

Registered nurses (RNs) are by far the largest professional healthcare group in the country. Approximately two million of them work in various specialties. Several of these specialties are described in detail in this chapter. Others are described in Part II. RNs are the most skilled and highly trained of nurses.

PREREQUISITES

Because nurses experience high physical and psychological stress on a continuing basis through direct contact with trauma and emergency situations, emotional stability is an essential characteristic for success. Patients in hospitals and nursing homes require 24-hour care, which means that some nurses work nights, weekends, and holidays. Nurses need considerable physical stamina for the extensive walking, standing, and patient-moving their jobs require. Nurses are exposed to a number of infectious diseases, among them AIDS, hepatitis, and tuberculosis, as well as to radiation, chemicals, and anesthetics. They must be able to accept responsibility, supervise others, follow orders precisely (but also be able to act independently when it is in the best interest of the patient to do so), and determine when further consultation is needed.

Finally, nurses should be caring and sympathetic. They take time to reassure worried patients and boost patient morale. Nurses are taught to recognize and understand patient needs and to provide emotional support as well as physical care. Often they take time to play with a child, read to a blind person, or write letters for a patient with a broken arm. Nurses help patients learn to function with disabilities or illness and teach patients how to take care of themselves after they are discharged from the hospital. Some nurses also care for newborn babies.

PREPARATION

All states require graduation from an accredited nursing school and successful completion of a national licensing exam. There are three principal educational routes to nursing:

1) ***Associate degrees in nursing*** *(A.D.N.) are offered by community and junior colleges, and take about two years. Approximately 60 percent of nursing school graduates come from A.D.N. programs. A few A.D.N. graduates become clinical nurse managers (formerly called head nurses) one of the few advancement positions available to them.*

2) ***Bachelor of science degrees in nursing*** *(B.S.N.), offered by colleges and universities, usually take four years. More than 30 percent of graduates come from these programs. The B.S.N. is a prerequisite for admission to graduate nursing programs. Those interested in research, consulting, teaching, or clinical specialization must enroll in a B.S.N. program. Some hospitals require staff nurses to have a B.S.N. degree.*

3) ***Diploma programs***, *given in hospitals, last two to three years. Less than 10 percent of the graduates in nursing come from these programs, a figure that is declining. In some instances, a diploma program will qualify graduates for a management position, although most such promotions are offered to RNs with a bachelor's or master's degree.*

Associate Degree Nursing Curriculum
Career Preparation in Two Years

FIRST YEAR

First Semester	Credits
Intro. to Human Nutrition	3
Human Development	3
Human Anatomy and Physiology	4
Fundamentals of Nursing	6
Physical Education	1
	17

Second Semester	Credits
English 1 or English Elective	3
Human Development	3
Human Anatomy and Physiology	4
Fundamentals of Nursing	6
	16

SECOND YEAR

First Semester	Credits
Approved Elective	3
Sociology	3
Nursing Care of Children and Adults	10
	16

Second Semester	Credits
Elective	3
Nursing Seminar	2
Nursing Care of Children and Adults	10
	15

For all three programs, education includes classroom instruction and supervised training in hospitals and other health facilities. Students in four-year programs take courses in anatomy, physiology, microbiology, chemistry, nutrition, psychology, and nursing. The two-year program is less rigorous academically, as you can see by the curriculum table above. Supervised clinical experience is provided in hospital departments such as pediatrics, psychiatry, maternity, and surgery.

Management-level nursing positions generally require a graduate degree in nursing or health services administration. According to the American Nurses Association, 43 percent of all nurses with master's degrees focused their graduate work on clinical practice. About 70 percent of those nurses with Ph.D.s, however, were involved in either education or research.

A good information source for educational financial aid programs is *Scholarships & Loans for Nursing Education,* an annually updated directory published by the National League for Nursing, 350 Hudson Street, New York, NY 10014. It includes tips on choosing a school, information about grant and other funding programs, and the best ways to apply for aid. For other information about financial assistance, see the Bibliography.

PRINCIPAL DUTIES

About two thirds of all employed registered nurses work in hospitals, almost 70 percent of them full-time. Most are staff nurses, who provide bedside nursing care and carry out the medical treatment prescribed by the physicians. They also may supervise licensed practical nurses (see page 38) and nursing aides (see page 156). Hospital nurses usually choose to specialize in one area of nursing, such as general medicine, surgery, maternity, emergency care, or intensive care. Some do "pool nursing," i.e., they rotate among departments on a periodic basis.

Nursing home nurses care for residents with conditions ranging from fractures to strokes. They assess each resident's condition, develop treatment plans, and supervise licensed practical nurses and nursing aides. They also work in specialty care environments, such as long-term rehabilitation for head injury patients or for patients with Alzheimer's disease.

Private duty nurses care for patients needing constant attention in patients' homes. They work directly for patients on a contract basis, or for a nursing employment agency that assigns them. (Agencies also provide private duty nurses on a temporary basis to some hospitals, nursing homes, and rehabilitation centers.) Other nurses are hired by stores or factories, or work in the armed forces.

OUTLOOK

According to the Bureau of Labor Statistics, about 20 percent of the 3.8 million new jobs in healthcare occupations will go to registered nurses. Employment of registered nurses is expected to grow much faster than the average of all occupations through the year 2005.

Employment in physicians' offices and clinics, including HMOs and emergency medical centers, is expected to grow rapidly—more so than in hospitals. More and more sophisticated procedures are being performed these days in non-hospital settings, largely because of accelerating advances in technology.

EARNINGS

The median annual earnings of full-time salaried registered nurses averages about $35,200, with some variations by geography and work setting. The bottom 10 percent earn almost $22,000, the top 10 percent a little over $50,000. For clinical nurse managers, the median is about $50,500; for clinical nurse specialists, it is almost $75,000. Other incentives, such as flexible work schedules, child care, educational benefits, and bonuses are becoming more prevalent for nurses.

> Resources:
> American Association of Colleges of Nursing
> 1 Dupont Circle, Suite 530
> Washington, DC 20036
>
> American Nurses' Association
> 600 Maryland Ave., SW
> Washington, DC 20024–2571

NURSE PRACTITIONER

Nurse practitioners (NPs) are registered nurses with an advanced education that expands their skills. In addition to basic nursing responsibilities, they perform many tasks formerly handled only by physicians.

PREREQUISITES

Nurse practitioners must be able to work independently and to manage stress well. An effective nurse practitioner is a true "people person" who thrives on a high degree of patient contact.

PREPARATION

To qualify for admission to a nurse practitioner program, all or most of the following are generally required: A baccalaureate degree in nursing, at least one year of professional nursing experience, satisfactory scores from either the Graduate Record Examination or the Miller Analogies Test, and undergraduate courses in statistics and research.

The nurse practitioner program is a master of science degree. Students take such courses as pharmacology, clinical applications of human physiology, health and illness appraisal, and clinical decision-making skills. Which certification examination one takes depends on whether a student has chosen an adult or family/pediatric track. Those wishing to specialize in adult care take the Adult Nurse Practitioner Certification examination. Those wishing to specialize in pediatrics take the Family Nurse Practitioner Certification examination.

PRINCIPAL DUTIES

Nurse practitioners work under the supervision of a licensed physician, often in a specialty such as pediatric or geriatric healthcare. Nurse practitioners provide direct patient care and perform physical examinations, diagnose illnesses, and administer and prescribe medications. They also take medical histories, order and interpret laboratory tests and x-rays, counsel patients, and, in some states, set simple fractures and suture minor wounds. NPs work in clinics, nursing homes, or hospitals.

Nurse Practitioners: A New Age in Healthcare

The American Nurses' Association stakes out a bold new role for nurse practitioners, particularly for the elderly, the poor, and those in underserved rural areas. Some of its conclusions:

- Some 60 to 80 percent of primary and preventive care traditionally done by doctors can be done by nurses for less money.
- Current restrictions on scope of practice, prescriptive authority, and eligibility for reimbursement severely impair nurse practitioners' ability to expand their roles.
- A Gallup poll shows 86 percent of the public willing to accept nurse practitioners as everyday healthcare providers.
- Certified Registered Nurse Anesthetists today are the sole providers of anesthetics in 85 percent of rural hospitals.
- In 1990, Certified Nurse-Midwives delivered 148,728 babies, about 3.6 percent of all U.S. births that year.

OUTLOOK

As healthcare reform in the United States continues into the twenty-first century, nurses will become a major force in designing and implementing new models of care for those in need. Nurse practitioners in particular are expected to be in high demand to provide both health maintenance and sick care services. The growing emphasis on public health, in which a number of nurse practitioners work, indicates yet another area of job opportunity potential.

EARNINGS

The median annual salary for a nurse practitioner is just under $47,500.

For information about nurse practitioners working as certified registered nurse anesthetists, see Chapter 4, Pursuing Careers in Anesthesiology.

Resource: **American Academy of Nurse Practitioners**
P.O. Box 12846
Austin, TX 78711

Computers and Nursing: Getting Your Career Online

Although personal computers are common at home and on campus, they are completely different from those used in hospitals.

Computers using medical software and computerized patient charts are in development nationwide. (Depending on where nurses had their training, their initial exposure to an automated chart may be on their first job.)

A medical office or clinic may use the computer for appointment scheduling and billing purposes only. Hospitals may also use the computer for communicating between departments, and for ordering tests, charging supplies, and automating the patient's chart.

An automated chart may include the entry and automatic graphing of vital signs and other diagnostic results, medication, intravenous charting, nurse's notes, retrieval of patient data, and care planning.

NURSE-MIDWIFE

Nurse-midwifery as a profession has gone far beyond its original function of "catching babies." Certified nurse-midwives (CNMs) now can provide primary health care for women, including comprehensive gynecologic and maternity care. More and more women are choosing CNMs for their maternity cycle care, from preconception and prenatal through labor and delivery to postpartum care.

PREREQUISITES

Nurse-midwifery focuses not just on physical care for the (expectant) mother and her baby but on the emotional needs of the entire family throughout the total period of involvement. Thus nurse-midwives must be accomplished obstetric professionals, to be sure; but they must be responsive, empathic, and intuitive, as well.

PREPARATION

A nurse-midwife must first be licensed as a registered nurse. Some nurse-midwifery education programs accept RNs with a diploma obtained through a hospital program. As an RN, you can then apply for admission to one of the seven certificate programs or 37 master's degree programs offered at medical centers and universities nationwide. (Several doctoral programs also are available.) Completion of these programs entitles the graduate to take the national examination to become a Certified Nurse-Midwife. The certificate program takes 9 to 12 months to complete; the master's program takes 16 to 24 months.

PRINCIPAL DUTIES

The care provided by certified nurse-midwives encompasses all of the essential factors of primary healthcare such as evaluation, assessment, treatment, and referral. CNMs work in hospitals, birth centers, private practices, health maintenance programs, clinics, universities, and homes. CNMs conduct physical examinations; identify health problems and make diagnoses; counsel women about nutrition, health habits, and other behaviors that can affect their pregnancy; provide physical and emotional support during labor; perform and repair episiotomies; repair lacerations; and administer medication and anesthesia to relieve pain. They provide postpartum care such as assessing infant health and nutritional needs, counseling new mothers on infant care, and prescribing medications and treatments as necessary.

OUTLOOK

About 4,500 nurse-midwives practice in the United States. The stated goal of the American College of Nurse-Midwives is to have 10,000 CNMs by the year 2001, so, as they say in their literature: "We want to hear from you." Lower cost and the trend toward insurance reimbursement for nurse-midwife assistance, as well as a growing trend toward natural childbirth, will keep interest high.

EARNINGS

Average salary for a certified nurse-midwife is about $57,500, with salaries over $75,000 in some locations for experienced CNMs.

    Resource: The American College of Nurse-Midwives
                         818 Connecticut Avenue NW, Suite 900
                         Washington, DC 20006
                         (career and educational information)

Nurse-Midwife Threat to Physicians

The idea that midwives are trying to wrest control of patient care from physicians, and jeopardizing the health of mothers and babies, was driven home by Dr. Kenneth J. Leaven, director of obstetrics at Parkland Memorial Hospital in Dallas, in a masterpiece of macho imagery. "It's sort of like putting a pilot who flies a Piper Cub in a 747," he said of midwives who take on complex cases. "When patients get into the airplane, they need to be told who's in the pilot's seat."

—*American Journal of Nursing* (July 1995)

LICENSED PRACTICAL NURSE

A licensed practical nurse (LPN) is to a registered nurse roughly what a physician assistant is to a physician. Many of the duties of the two overlap, but the responsibilities are not as heavy and the education and licensing procedures are not as rigorous for the LPN. Consequently, the paychecks for licensed practical nurses are not as large as they are for registered nurses.

PREREQUISITES

Like most other kinds of nurses, LPNs (or LVNs, for licensed vocational nurses, as they are known in some states) should have a caring, sympathetic nature. Their occupational hazards are similar to those of the RN, including long days on their feet and the stress of working with sick patients and their families. Those LPNs employed in nursing homes—an increasing number because of our aging population—face patients who may be confused, irrational, or uncooperative.

PRINCIPAL DUTIES

LPNs provide basic bedside care. They take vital signs, treat bedsores, apply dressings, give alcohol rubs and massages, apply ice packs and hot water bottles, and insert catheters. *Medical* LPNs, who have completed additional coursework in pharmacology, are allowed to prepare and give injections, administer prescribed medicines, and start intravenous fluids. Some help deliver and care for infants. Experienced LPNs may supervise nursing assistants and aides.

OUTLOOK

Job prospects for LPNs are expected to be excellent. The number of new graduates needed will be well above that of recent years. Very rapid growth is expected in such residential care facilities as board-and-care homes, nursing homes, and group homes for the mentally retarded, as well as in home healthcare services. LPNs hold about 700,000 jobs.

EARNINGS

Median annual earnings for salaried LPNs is approximately $23,400. The bottom 10 percent earn a little more than $16,300; the top 10 percent earn more than $33,000. Median figures for LPNs working in nursing homes is a little less.

    Resource: **National Federation of Licensed Practical Nurses**
                             P.O. Box 18088
                             Raleigh, NC 27619

ANOTHER WAY TO GET THERE

Peter Leighton, CNA (not his real name), decided on a nursing career only after trying tree surgery, gas station attendant, galley hand, ship steward, waiter, chef, bartender, night club manager, and non-profit business manager. Below, he traces his circuitous career path:

After high school, all I had in mind was to make money—as much and as fast as I could. I realized that working in gas stations and as a tree surgeon were not going to do it, so I got a job as a galley hand on an offshore oil rig. The beauty of that kind of work is that you save everything you make. You're paid for 84 hours a week and you're away as much as six months at a time, so you can save a lot of money.

I made beds, washed dishes—anything the steward asked me to do. Not long after that I was promoted to night cook, and then a year later to steward. We fed all three crews, so there were meals to make 24 hours a day.

With some of my savings I bought part interest in a night club, which was very successful. Later I got into the restaurant business, which was also successful.

But something was missing. I wanted work with more substance—something more gratifying. In 1980 or so, I took a part-time job with Goodwill Industries in Bridgeport supervising the sheltered workshop. It paid terribly. The employees were mostly mentally or emotionally handicapped and subsidized by the state. They couldn't make more than $60 a month without getting penalized for it, but most weren't making anywhere near that. It wasn't long before two other positions opened up there, one of which was Rehabilitation Manager. In that position I came up with a time-study plan and arranged for more specialized responsibilities. This encouraged everyone to make more money.

Eventually I realized that something had to give. I was working four jobs and my marriage was falling apart. A job opened up with the City of Bridgeport, coordinating the office for persons with disabilities—an advocacy agency. It was very rewarding and well paying, but I burned out after about two years because of the caseload. Where it had been 50 to 60 at Goodwill, it was 150 at the disability agency.

I had just decided to go back to the restaurant—they made me a great offer—when my dad got sick. I was the only one in the immediate family not married or with children at the time, so I agreed to do it, and worked out a schedule where I could handle both the job and my father. For three years I drove 15 miles to New Canaan in the morning, got him up, fed him, bathed him, gave him his medication, put him down for his nap, and then drove back to the restaurant in time for the lunch customers.

I'd work there 'til two, and drive back to get my dad up from his nap, clean him, feed him, and take him for a ride. By this time my mother would be home, so I'd make dinner for them and go home.

I had never gotten along with my dad, but this became a period of catharsis for both of us. We rediscovered each other, and our relationship was much better than it had been when I was growing up. And these were not ideal circumstances. Think of the role reversal. A parent accustomed to being caretaker is suddenly the one being cared for. For this to have happened—with dignity—was extremely difficult for both of us.

Eventually, of course, my dad died. But I realized what I wanted to do with my life. This my dad gave me. I enrolled in nursing courses for my associate's degree at a community college, and was certified as a nurse's assistant in 1993.

The Sunday after graduation I saw two ads in the paper. I sent my résumé and a cover letter, and was offered both jobs! The one I chose was perfect. This was a man who had been in cardiac arrest and was traumatically brain injured—totally deprived of oxygen for 12 minutes. He was gone—saw the white light and everything.

He is an accomplished author—17 books—and even with his brain injury he has an I.Q. of 126. He also invented the first personal computer, by the way, which is now in a Boston computer museum.

In three and a half years this family had had 11 nurses. So in my first job I was put into a situation where the patient's interests are so scattered—he needs entertainment continuously—that I had to be in four different places at one time and never leave the room.

He's only fifty-two, and the doctors say he's never going to get any better. That's not his view, of course, and I try to reinforce his optimism any way I can. I take him to his doctor's appointments, and I've met all his physicians. I see what the eye therapists do, for example, and we repeat some of the same exercises at home. He hadn't been out of his wheelchair for six years, so therapy of many kinds was really important. Like he'll stand in front of me while I have him in a bear hug, and I nudge him behind his knees with my knees to keep his legs going. He thinks he's going to walk again, which is fine.

My job is to be sure his health needs are provided for. If I can make his life more meaningful, then it doesn't matter how unrealistic his dreams are. I think empathy means just as much as training in this job. It's not for everybody. You have to sit down and evaluate the patient's needs, and then figure out how you can fulfill them. It's wonderful to be able to provide a foundation for someone who has been secure all his life and then had it taken away—and now after 11 nurses to have one he can depend on.

The pay is excellent—much more, I know, than a CNA who works in a hospital. It's insurance reimbursed, which is unusual working out of a home. And I get a raise every year.

In the three years I've been there, every day is different. It's exciting. The point is, if you see someone else happy, you're going to be happy.

NURSE EXECUTIVE

The nursing executive track prepares nurses to become nurse managers and administrators. There are two administrative nursing roles:

1) **Nurse executives** *are RNs who are part of healthcare management. With titles such as vice president or chief operating officer, nurse executives are responsible for quality, cost-effective patient-care delivery in the entire hospital.*
2) **Nurse managers** *are RNs who are members of middle management. With titles such as clinical nurse manager, unit manager, or director, nurse managers are responsible 24 hours a day for operations and patient care delivery on one or more patient care units.*

PREREQUISITES

Nursing executives must be good managers, able to hire and train employees for maximum contribution to the department or institution. They must be creative problem-solvers, and bring projects in on schedule and to budget. They should have an awareness of and be able to apply basic principles of quality control.

PREPARATION

A nurse executive program leads to a master of science degree. Requirements for consideration are similar to those for a nurse practitioner program. Students in a nursing executive program take courses with such titles as "Nursing and Change in Healthcare Services," "Administrative Theories in Nursing," "Resource and Financial Management," "Financial Management for Clinicians," and "Healthcare Planning."

PRINCIPAL DUTIES

Nurse executives are responsible for overseeing the smooth functioning of the department, division, or hospital they supervise. They lead and motivate staff members, hire and fire staff, and ensure that patient standards are met.

OUTLOOK

The number of nurse executives continues to increase as more RNs move into positions previously occupied by hospital administrators.

EARNINGS

Average base salary nationwide is $91,800. Salaries range from $46,000 to $200,000. On average, men ($100,000) earn slightly more than women ($91,000).

Resource: **American Organization of Nurse Executives**
840 North Lake Shore Drive
Chicago, IL 60611

PART II

Career Opportunities Within Specialties

The following 15 chapters cover medical career opportunities
representing a wide range of interests and need.
Content decisions were made partly to reflect current or evolving
practice, and may shift further within the next year or two.
Please refer to specific sources
mentioned for the most up-to-date figures.

CHAPTER 4

Pursuing Careers in Anesthesiology

Years ago anyone undergoing an operation was given "gas"—often ether or chloroform—to induce artificial sleep. Thus the pain was blocked, as intended, but often the patient awoke to violent stomach cramps, vomiting, and extreme pain when the anesthesia wore off.

Today patients need not wake up nauseated and in pain. Many have the option not only of remaining completely conscious throughout their procedures but of watching the details on a nearby television monitor. In other surgeries, regional pain blocks, administered into the spinal fluid or just outside the spinal column, keep patients pain free.

Even in cases requiring general anesthesia, risks are far lower than they used to be for the more than 26 million people undergoing some form of anesthesia each year. Recent advances in patient monitoring have sharply reduced the occasional oxygen starvation that used to cause brain damage and heart attacks (for which reason anesthesiologists for a time had the highest malpractice insurance rates of all classifications of physicians). Newer anesthetic drugs are safer and have fewer side effects, as well.

ANESTHESIOLOGIST

In 1992, the American Medical Association rated anesthesiologists among the most highly paid of all specializing physicians, a status intact for at least a decade. Since that time their remuneration seems to have peaked, for several reasons: (1) Their high salaries have come under increasing scrutiny by cost-conscious hospital and health management organization administrators (to the benefit of more modestly compensated nurse anesthetists—see page 46). (2) Medical students opted to specialize in anesthesiology in record numbers, resulting in an oversupply of anesthesiologists. (3) Widely quoted studies have suggested that many once-common procedures requiring anesthesia—hysterectomies, angioplasties, and middle-ear tube insertions, for example—are of uncertain benefit.

The result has been a largely market-driven squeeze on anesthesiology. HMOs and other managed-care plans have reduced surgery and hospitalization rates for members. This unexpectedly low growth rate in surgery has translated to less business for anesthesiologists. Consequently, charges for anesthesia services are falling. Even Medicare, traditionally a big source of anesthesiologist income, has tightened considerably.

PREREQUISITES

An ability to anticipate problems and then solve them is a definite asset for anyone interested in anesthesiology. Because of the variety of sophisticated, space-age equipment in use, anesthesiologists must also have sharp critical thinking skills to efficiently oversee the multiple monitors and alarms in use during the operation. In emergency situations they must have the ability to counteract cardiopulmonary and respiratory care problems, as well as manage critically ill and/or injured patients. Finally, the anesthesiologist is directly responsible for patient cooperation and demeanor. An operation is serious business. The tension it creates in the patient must be acknowledged, isolated, and neutralized to assure a minimum number of distracting elements for the surgeon to deal with. Having a good bedside manner as a requisite skill takes on another dimension.

PREPARATION

A minimum of four years of graduate medical education is necessary to train a physician who intends to specialize in anesthesiology. Three of these years must be in clinical anesthesia. One of the four years is a "clinical base year," providing the resident with 12 months of clinical education in medical disciplines other than the administration of anesthesia. Instruction during the clinical base year includes content in internal medicine, pediatrics, surgery, obstetrics, gynecology, neurology, family practice, or any combination of these specialties. The other three years consist of training in basic anesthesia, subspecialty anesthesia, and advanced anesthesia.

PRINCIPAL DUTIES

Whereas the surgeon's work in the operating theater starts after the patient is asleep, the anesthesiologist's responsibility begins as soon as the patient is wheeled into the room, and often even earlier, with a preoperative appointment to review medical history and deal with apprehensions. A claustrophobic patient, for example, may be fearful of the mask used to administer anesthesia. The anesthesiologist will either relieve these fears or decide to use another method. Sometimes a patient who easily becomes nauseated is given preventive medication. Those patients with a need for emotional or psychological control may be difficult to deal with during an operation and require counseling to minimize any possible disturbances.

During the operation, the anesthesiologist is the team member who monitors blood pressure, pulse, heartbeat, and other vital signs. There are seven to ten drugs that may adversely interact with the body's chemical balance. Many tests are administered to the patient beforehand to anticipate any adverse reactions, of course, but during the surgery not everything can be expected to go as smoothly as programmed. Complications are uncommon, but no anesthetic procedure is without risk. Occasionally the anesthesiologist must deal with an irregular heartbeat, low blood pressure, or allergic reactions.

The anesthesiologist or nurse anesthetist is also there when the patient awakes, and is on call to deal with any situations that may arise during the two hours or so of grogginess that most patients experience after coming out of anesthesia.

The Power of Positive Suggestion

Anesthesiology professor James C. Erickson II recommended in *Prevention* magazine that positive suggestions become a part of anesthesia. He found that patients who receive positive suggestions, such as the sharing of optimistic prognoses from members of the surgical team, leave the recovery room faster than expected.

OUTLOOK

Because of factors mentioned at the beginning of this chapter, the short-term future for this country's 32,000 anesthesiologists is flat, at best. A study prepared by Abt Associates, a Maryland consulting firm, revealed that in many areas of the country there may be twice as many anesthesiologists as needed. The Abt study noted that for many procedures, nurse anesthetists could be used in place of the more highly trained, better-paid doctors.

EARNINGS

Because of growing market saturation, as well as several other factors previously noted, salaries for anesthesiologists will likely level off. Add to this the fact that charges for anesthesia services are tumbling in many areas, and it becomes apparent that their earnings can go in only one direction. Between 1982 and 1992 the average annual earnings for anesthesiologists increased by 73 percent, from $132,000 to $228,500. During the next ten years this figure probably will fall back closer to the 1982 level.

    Resource: American Society of Anesthesiologists
                       520 N. Northwest Highway
                       Park Ridge, IL 60068
                       (career path and education information)

NURSE ANESTHETIST

Certified registered nurse anesthetists (CRNAs) are the principal beneficiaries of the backlash affecting anesthesiologists. First of all, most make less than half as much money per year as their physician counterparts. This makes an attractive alternative for hospital and HMO administrators anxious to reduce costs. CRNAs are advanced-practice nurses. This being so, nursing statutes do not require a nurse anesthetist to be supervised by an anesthesiologist. CRNAs administer anesthesia in all 50 states, and are legally authorized to administer every kind of anesthetic care.

PREREQUISITES

The skills required and personality traits desired for CRNAs are identical to those for anesthesiologists.

EDUCATION

A CRNA must have a bachelor's degree, current license as a registered nurse, and a strong clinical background in acute/critical care nursing before completing a minimum of two years of graduate level education in anesthesiology. CRNAs and anesthesiologists take the same Advanced Cardiac Life Support Certification course. CRNAs also must continually demonstrate their ability in their specialty through recertification programs every two years.

Military Nurse Anesthetist Remembers V-J Day

At a 1991 50th anniversary of V-J Day celebration, Annie Mealer, an army nurse anesthetist from Walter Reed Hospital, recalled her first assignment, at Corregidor Hospital in the Philippines, with her staff of 12 nurses and 500 patients:

After the bombing of Pearl Harbor we were ordered to set up a hospital section in Malinta Tunnel. There were only a couple of water spigots for the entire hospital, and no toilet facilities. The electricians worked on the lights and ventilating system....

Christmas, 1941. The air-raid signal went off, and we only had time to jump into a ditch. It sounded as if the whole world were being blown away. The Japanese bombs missed very little on the island that day.... We were rushed to the tunnel in a car between waves of bombs. In the tunnel I threw my helmet off, tied my hair up in a piece of gauze, and checked the shock wards to see if they had adequate help. Then to the operating room, where I gave anesthetics to one casualty after another....

As the days passed, the bombing intensified. The shelling and bombing was so constant we did not dare go near the tunnel entrance. I was working daily from 12 to 14 hours in the operating room....

I was called to the commanding officer's office and told they were evacuating the nurses; a group would leave that night. I was to be ready. I turned and walked out. When I reached the main tunnel, I heard a voice call, "Clear the way for casualties." I looked at the face on the litter as it passed....

I went back to the operating room. As I sat administering anesthesia, I reviewed the cases in the tunnel. They all needed help that only a nurse could give them. I sent word to my CO [Commanding Officer] that I would stay with them. Here in this tunnel choked with shell smoke and misery was a group of people that meant more to me than anything else."

Annie Mealer was taken prisoner when Corregidor fell to the Japanese. She was released from prison by American troops in February, 1945, and was later awarded the Philippine Defense Ribbon for her wartime bravery.

PRINCIPAL DUTIES

In most instances, CRNAs perform the same duties as anesthesiologists. Most exceptions occur in team situations, when an anesthesiologist supervises the work of one or more nurse anesthetists. In either case, working independently or with an anesthesiologist, CRNAs administer more than 65 percent of all anesthetics given patients each year.

OUTLOOK

The American Association of Nurse Anesthetists represents more than 25,000 CRNAs nationwide. Currently there is a shortage of nurse anesthetists, with studies indicating a continuing need at least until the year 2005.

EARNINGS

The average salary of a nurse anesthetist rose more than 50 percent from 1987 to 1992, from $53,000 to $82,700, according to an AANA survey. Compensation can go up to $140,000 for independent contractors.

Resource: American Association of Nurse Anesthetists
             222 South Prospect Avenue
             Park Ridge, IL 60068
             (career path and educational information)

ANOTHER WAY TO GET THERE

James L. Hawes is an Iowa CRNA whose training and career was jump-started by the U.S. Navy. In addition to a full nursing schedule he is also a counselor on the online service CompuServe for others thinking about nurse anesthetist careers. Here's how it all came about, in Jim's words:

As a child growing up in Atlantic, Iowa, I had only two aspirations: to be either a veterinarian or a teacher. Actually, my first dream was to be a surgeon, like my uncle in Mesa, Arizona, or a small town doctor like my grandfather. I guess I was influenced too much by those around me who said I wasn't smart enough to be a doctor. So early on I worked with a blacksmith helping to shoe horses, and at a saddle shop in town.

Then in high school I needed a better paying job, and my mother suggested I apply at the local hospital as a nurse's aide. She was a registered nurse there—and probably my greatest motivational guide. I wasn't happy about it, but the job was better than I thought it would be. I was given duties only nurses in city hospitals get. Being one of only two male aides at the hospital, I was quite a novelty. (The two of us were even written up in the town paper.) It was at that point that nursing as a profession began to appeal to me.

I decided to break down the females-only barrier. When I graduated from high school I moved to Omaha, Nebraska, and found a job at a large city hospital. It was there that I saw how much further I could go with a degree—and decided to get one. The first school I applied to turned me down—because I was male! The next one accepted me, but it closed after only a year and a half, unfortunately. At that point I decided to join the navy. My recruiter, seeing that I had nearly two years of nursing school, advised me to finish up, and then join as an officer. That sounded good to me. With the navy's help I found another school in Omaha, finished the program successfully, and was commissioned an ensign in the Navy Nurse Corps in 1969.

My navy experience was an excellent learning and motivational tool. I quickly realized that I needed to specialize in an advanced nursing practice, and remembered a day as a junior nursing student during surgery rotation. A CRNA called me over to her station and demonstrated the delivery of anesthesia. I was fascinated—and after a half-hour I was hooked.

Actually, this attraction might go back even further. At ages five and twelve I had surgery at a small rural hospital. The CRNA was a big woman with a kind heart, and I'll always remember what she did for me. I wasn't afraid at all, thanks to her. Both times she let me watch her preparations, and I was entranced.

I enjoy being a CRNA because I help patients through a very stressful time in their lives, and I also help the surgeons do their job. The long hours and down-time can be frustrating, but a successful anesthetic is always worth the effort. I have worked both with and without anesthesiologists, and for the most part I like having their medical knowledge to fall back on. I have run into only a few who were unbearable. I guess you could say it's a good character builder.

I think CRNAs will have a very valuable place in this country well into the next century, expecially in rural and county hospitals. CRNAs have lost some autonomy in city hospitals, but we just need to keep proving that we are well trained and necessary.

If I were to become a nurse again, there's no doubt I would choose anesthesiology as my specialty.

ANESTHESIOLOGIST ASSISTANT

In 1975 the American Society of Anesthesiologists sanctioned a new profession, designed to answer a need for anesthetists with technical backgrounds. Today approximately 500 anesthesiologist assistants (AAs) work in the field.

PREREQUISITES

Because AAs work with patients under the direction of anesthesiologists, the skills and demeanor required roughly mirror those of anesthesiologists.

PREPARATION

Qualification for the two-year master's degree program includes a premed bachelor's degree. Although any major is acceptable (if premed requirements are met), the most desirable courses are biology, chemistry, physics, mathematics, computer science, or one of the allied health professions—such as respiratory therapy, or medical technology—or nursing. Currently, the only two colleges offering AA programs are Emory University, in Atlanta, Georgia, and Case-Western Reserve University, in Cleveland, Ohio.

PRINCIPAL DUTIES

Anesthesiologist assistants are roughly analagous to physician assistants (see page 27) as far as their responsibilities are concerned. AAs also assist the anesthesiologist (or in some cases the nurse anesthetist) in collecting preoperative data, such as taking health histories, inserting intravenal and arterial catheters, and administering drugs for induction and maintenance of anesthesia.

OUTLOOK

The future for AAs is likely to be better than that for anesthesiologists but not quite as good as for nurse anesthetists because they are neither as skilled nor as versatile. They are in greatest need in medium and large hospitals, where the incidence of complex cases with more extensive patient monitoring (cardiac surgery, neurosurgery, transplant surgery, and the like) is prevalent.

EARNINGS

Salaries vary depending on skill level and years of experience, with $60,000 to $70,000 being an average entry-level range for a 40-hour work week, plus benefits.

Resources: American Academy of Anesthesiologists' Assistants
P.O. Box 33876
Decatur, GA 30033-0876
(career and education information)

Accreditation Review Committee for the
 Anesthesiologist Assistant
7108-C South Alton Way
Englewood, CO 80112
(program and accreditation information)

CHAPTER 5

Pursuing Careers in Cardiovascular Medicine

Many U.S. cities maintain a healthcare information line, sponsored by local hospitals and other providers to maintain communication with residents, as well as to provide them with a way to qualify symptoms of possible health problems against medical definitions, by specialty. In many instances one dials the appropriate number from a Yellow Pages "Physicians and Surgeons" or "Hospitals" listing, and punches in a three- or four-digit code for a taped message in the special area requested. Here is one typical message, programmed to offer basic cardiac information:

"The heart has four components: (1) vessels that carry blood to nourish the heart muscle; (2) the muscle itself, which is responsible for pumping blood to the body; (3) valves, which direct the blood flow; and (4) the heart's nervous system, which tells the heart when to pump. Heart trouble can be caused by any one of these components.

"For example, when the blood vessels of the heart are affected by coronary artery disease, the blood flow to the muscle is diminished, and a heart attack may occur. Or, if the valves are affected by heart disease, they may block the blood flow to the heart or leak the blood backward, and heart failure may occur. The most common causes of valve problems are rheumatic fever, birth defects, or damage to the valve from heart attacks. Finally, if the heart's nervous system fails, a condition called an arrhythmia can result. This is a disorder affecting the regularity—or rhythm—of the heartbeat. Arrhythmia causes the heart to beat too quickly, too slowly, or in irregular fashion. If untreated, these rhythm disturbances can be dangerous.

"These are the basic types of heart disease."

Through such community efforts, awareness is kept at a high level in most parts of the country about these and other healthcare issues. It is then up to the professionals in the various specialties to respond to specific needs. Here are some of the cardiovascular specialists who face such problems daily.

CARDIOLOGIST

Also called heart specialists, cardiologists diagnose and treat diseases of the heart, using medical instruments and specialized equipment. They study diagnostic images and electrocardiograph recordings to aid in making diagnoses. They prescribe medications, and recommend dietary and activity programs, as needed. They also refer patients to surgeons specializing in cardiac cases when a need for corrective surgery is indicated, and engage in research to study the anatomy of, and diseases peculiar to, the heart.

Cardiologists provide for the continuing care of heart patients. They supervise all aspects of therapy, including the administration of drugs to modify heart functions.

Cardiologists must be able to diagnose and treat such acute and chronic cardiovascular conditions as congestive heart failure, acute myocardial infarction (heart attack), hypertension, valvular and pulmonary heart disease, infections and inflammatory heart disease, and adult congenital heart disease. Their specialty training program usually lasts three years, after the completion of all educational requirements for physicians described in Chapter 2, Career Opportunities as Doctors. Career outlook and earnings prospects for cardiologists also are covered in Chapter 2.

CARDIOVASCULAR TECHNOLOGIST

The American Medical Association Council on Medical Education officially recognized cardiovascular technology as an allied health profession in 1981. Cardiovascular technologists perform diagnostic examinations at the request of a physician. They then create data from which a patient's correct anatomic and physiologic diagnosis may be established.

PREREQUISITES

Cardiovascular technologists must be reliable, have excellent mechanical aptitude, and be able to follow detailed instructions. A pleasant, relaxed manner for putting patients at ease is also an asset.

PREPARATION

Cardiovascular technologists must complete a two-year community or technical college program. One year is devoted to core courses, followed by a year of specialized instruction in either invasive, noninvasive, or noninvasive peripheral cardiology. Those qualified in a related allied health profession need to complete only one year of specialized education.

PRINCIPAL DUTIES

Cardiovascular technologists who specialize in cardiac catheterization procedures, also known as invasive technology, are called cardiology technologists. They assist a physician who winds a small tube, or catheter, through a patient's blood vessel from the leg into the heart to determine if a blockage exists, and for other diagnostic purposes. Cardiovascular technologists may also specialize in noninvasive peripheral vascular tests. They use ultrasound equipment that transmits sound waves, then collects the echoes to form an image on a screen. Some cardiovascular technologists schedule appointments, type doctor's interpretations, maintain patients' files, and care for equipment.

OUTLOOK

Job outlook in this field is expected to grow faster than the average for all occupations for the next several years. Growth will occur as the population ages, because older people have a higher incidence of heart problems.

EARNINGS

According to the American Society for Cardiovascular Professionals, average salary for cardiovascular technologists is about $32,000 annually. Cardiovascular technologists specializing in echocardiography earn between $21,000 and $33,000; cardiac catheterization technologists can earn up to $34,000.

> Resource: **American Society for Cardiovascular Professionals**
> 10500 Wakeman Drive
> Fredericksburg, VA 22407

EKG TECHNICIAN

EKG (for electrocardiogram) technicians administer tests that trace electrical impulses transmitted by the heart, such as Holter monitoring (explained below), and stress testing, to assist physicians in diagnosing and treating cardiac and blood vessel ailments.

PREREQUISITES

Same as for cardiovascular technologists, except that the equipment used is not quite as sophisticated or complex.

PREPARATION

For technicians using just basic EKGs, Holter monitoring, and stress testing, one-year programs still exist, although most EKG technicians are still trained on the job by an EKG supervisor or a cardiologist. Such training lasts 8 to 16 weeks, and candidates need a high school diploma to qualify.

PRINCIPAL DUTIES

To take a basic EKG, technicians attach electrodes to the patient's chest, arms, and legs, then manipulate switches on an electrocardiograph machine to get the reading. This test is done before most kinds of surgery and as part of a routine physical exam for older people.

For a Holter monitoring, technicians place electrodes on the patient's chest and attach a portable EKG monitor to the patient's belt. After 24 to 48 hours of normal routine for the patient, they remove a tape from the monitor, place it in a scanner, and send it to a physician.

For a treadmill stress-test, EKG technicians take a medical history, explain the procedure, connect the patient to an EKG monitor, and obtain a baseline reading and resting blood pressure. While the patient is on a treadmill, they then monitor the heart, gradually increasing the speed of the treadmill to observe the effect of increased exertion.

OUTLOOK

Employment of EKG technicians is expected to decline. Although the number of cardiac tests and procedures performed is anticipated to grow, demand for EKG technicians is not likely to keep pace because many hospitals are expected to train registered nurses and others to perform basic EKG procedures.

EARNINGS

Based on a 40-hour work week, the median annual salary for EKG technicians is a little under $18,000, with the average minimum a little under $16,000, and the average maximum almost $23,000.

Heartcare Breakthrough Chronology

Early 1900s	Digitalis is the first drug used to treat congestive heart failure by making the heart pump with more force.
1945	Anticoagulants are introduced to help prevent blood clots.
1947	Electric defibrillation, the use of an electric shock, is found to restore normal rhythm to a fibrillating heart.
1948	Cardiac catheterization, the process of advancing a thin tube (catheter) into a vein, artery, or heart chamber to perform diagnostic studies, is developed.
1952	Diuretics are approved for use in the treatment of congestive heart failure and high blood pressure to help the body eliminate excess salt and water.
1954	The heart-lung machine is developed. A mechanical pump oxygenates and pumps blood during heart surgery, making open-heart surgery possible.
1955	Cardiac massage becomes an accepted technique to revive an arrested heart.
1958	The first external pacemaker is used to pace a baby's heart after surgery.
1959	Three major classes of therapeutic drugs become available: beta blockers, nitrates, and antihypertensives.

1960 . . . . A pacemaker is successfully implanted. The first successful heart-valve replacement is performed with a mechanical valve.

1962 . . . . The intra-aortic balloon pump, which temporarily increases coronary artery blood flow, is introduced.

1968 . . . .
- Coronary angiography, which allows physicians to examine blood vessels or chambers of the heart by tracing the course of dye injected into the bloodstream, is introduced.
- Bypass surgery is developed. It improves the heart's blood supply by constructing a detour around the blocked part of the coronary artery with a blood vessel from another part of the body.
- The first heart transplant occurs.

1969 . . . . The first artificial heart implant takes place, used for three days before the transplant of a human heart.

1972 . . . . Antilipid drugs are introduced, to reduce the amount of serum cholesterol circulating in the blood.

1973 . . . . A genetic defect that raises blood cholesterol levels and causes coronary heart disease is discovered.

1974 . . . . Calcium channel blockers are used to lower blood pressure, reduce the frequency of angina attacks, and help prevent repeat heart attacks.

1977 . . . . Angioplasty, using balloons or lasers, is used to open an occluded coronary artery.

1980 . . . . ACE inhibitors are used to open constricted blood vessels.

1984 . . . . A large-scale human experiment proves that lowering blood cholesterol levels reduces the risk of a heart attack.

1985 . . . . The implantable defibrillator becomes available to restore normal rhythm to a fibrillating heart.

PERFUSIONIST

The field of cardiovascular perfusion emerged in the mid-1960s, with most practitioners trained on the job until the mid-1970s. They were originally called extra-corporeal technologists, meaning they operate circulation equipment during any medical situation where it is necessary to support or temporarily replace the patient's circulatory or respiratory function. Trainees often come from other disciplines: nursing, respiratory therapy, surgical technology, and the laboratory.

PREREQUISITES

Perfusionists need skilled hands, high mechanical aptitude, and good powers of concentration. Perfusionists work under highly stressful situations, and often must make snap decisions affecting the life of the patient. For this reason emotional stability is a crucial attribute.

PREPARATION

Perfusion programs vary in length from one year to 44 months, depending on program design, objectives, and student qualifications. Thirty-five programs are currently available in 21 states and the District of Columbia. Tuition costs can vary from $3,000 to $15,000 per year. (The difference is largely due to different tuition for residents and non-residents.) Curriculum courses include anatomy, physiology, chemistry, pharmacology, and heart-lung bypass preparation for both adults and children.

PRINCIPAL DUTIES

Perfusionists operate and monitor heart-lung machines essential in open-heart surgery, liver transplants, and cancer surgery, among other procedures. They must be able to quickly replace lost or lowered blood volume to minimize trauma. During cardiopulmonary bypass, the perfusionist may administer blood products, anesthetics, or drugs, and is responsible for purchasing supplies and equipment, as well as for personnel and departmental management.

OUTLOOK

Cardiovascular perfusion is a relatively new profesion. Only about 3,000 men and women work in the field today. Employment for perfusionists is expected to grow much faster than the average for all occupations over the next several years. As transplant technology improves and the number of bypass operations continues to increase at its present rate, the need for experienced perfusionists will increase steadily.

EARNINGS

New graduates from one of the perfusion programs can expect to earn $40,000 or more per year. The annual average for experienced perfusionists is from $50,000 to $80,000 annually. Some busy practitioners earn more than $100,000 a year.

Resources: **AmSECT National Office**
11480 Sunset Hills Road, Suite 200E
Reston, VA 22090
(career and curriculum information)

Accreditation Committee for Perfusion Education
7108-C at S. Alton Way
Englewood, CO 30112

RESPIRATORY THERAPIST

Respiratory therapy personnel are concerned with breathing disorders. They evaluate them, treat them, and care for patients who suffer from them. Many respiratory disorders stem from such ailments as pneumonia, chronic bronchitis, emphysema, and heart disease.

PREREQUISITES

Respiratory therapists should be sensitive to patients' physical and psychological needs. Respiratory care workers must pay attention to detail, follow instructions, and work as part of a team. Operating complicated respiratory therapy equipment requires mechanical ability and manual dexterity.

PREPARATION

Formal training is necessary to enter this field. Training is offered by hospitals, medical schools, colleges and universities, trade schools, vocational-technical institutes, and the armed forces. Some programs prepare graduates for jobs as respiratory therapists; other, shorter programs lead to jobs as respiratory therapy technicians.

High school students interested in a respiratory care career should take courses in mathematics, health, biology, chemistry, and physics. Thirty-seven states license respiratory care personnel. Two credentials are awarded to respiratory care practitioners who satisfy the requirements: Certified Respiratory Therapy Technician (CRTT) and Registered Respiratory Therapist (RRT). All graduates—those from two- and four-year programs in respiratory therapy, as well as those from one-year technician programs—may take the CRTT examination. CRTTs who meet education and experience requirements can take a separate examination, leading to an RRT.

PRINCIPAL DUTIES

Respiratory therapists treat a wide range of patients: premature infants whose lungs are not fully developed, elderly people with chronic asthma or emphysema, and people who need emergency care for heart failure, drowning, or shock. Respiratory therapists most commonly use oxygen or oxygen mixtures, chest physiotherapy, and aerosol medications. Therapists also connect patients who cannot breathe on their own to ventilators that deliver pressurized air into the lungs. They insert a tube into a patient's trachea (windpipe); connect the tube to the ventilator; and set the rate, volume, and oxygen concentration of the air entering the patient's lungs.

Respiratory therapists perform chest physiotherapy on patients to remove mucus from their lungs to make it easier for them to breathe. During surgery, for example, anesthesia depresses respiration, so this treatment may be prescribed to help get the patient's lungs back to normal and prevent congestion.

OUTLOOK

Employment of respiratory therapists and respiratory therapy technicians is expected to increase much faster than the average for all occupations over the next several years. The elderly are the most common sufferers from respiratory ailments. Because of an increasing population of middle-aged and older people, the incidence of pulmonary disease will likewise increase.

EARNINGS

Median annual earnings for respiratory therapists is a little over $32,000. The top 10 percent earned just over $48,000, and the bottom 10 percent just over $21,500. Entry-level therapists earn on average just under $25,000. Earnings for respiratory therapy technicians average $25,500 annually.

Resource: American Association for Respiratory Care
11030 Ables Lane
Dallas, TX 75229
(career and educational information)

CHAPTER 6
Pursuing Careers in Dentistry

Dentists care for their patients in many ways, but primarily by identifying, preventing, and correcting problems of the teeth and the tissues and nerves that support them. Modern dentistry began with the introduction of general anesthetics to relieve pain, during the mid-1800s. The widespread use of high-speed dental drills by the turn of the century further reduced pain, and with it some of the apprehension most people felt about "going to the dentist." It was at this point that dentistry began to emerge as a sought-after career.

DENTIST

Approximately 200,000 dentists now practice in the United States, about 90 percent of them as private practitioners. Their work goes far beyond the widely held perception that they either fill teeth or pull them. Actually, they are able to contribute significantly to the quality of their patients' day-to-day lives by preventing tooth decay and gum disease, and by treating and correcting various injuries and deformities of the neck, face, and jaw, as well as by performing root canals and other procedures.

PREREQUISITES

Men and women who pursue careers as dentists are generally motivated, scientifically curious, intelligent, ambitious, and socially conscious. Both manual dexterity and scientific ability are important to success. Dentists need skilled, steady hands, as well as a good sense of space and shape. In a profession highly dependent on contact with people, interpersonal skills are crucial.

The First Use of Ether

Dr. William Morton, a Massachusetts dentist, first used ether in a tooth extraction at the suggestion of Charles Jackson, a professor of chemistry at Harvard University. In 1846 Morton publicly demonstrated this concept in an operation performed at Massachusetts General Hospital. Follow-up publicity quickly led to the use of ether as an anesthetic in Britain and France, as well as in other countries.

In 1850 the French Academy of Science awarded the Montyon prize of 5,000 francs to Jackson and Morton jointly. Both men claimed sole credit, however, and Morton refused to share the prize. After a bitter quarrel and subsequent lawsuits, Morton was ruined financially.

PREPARATION

Prospective dental students should plan an academic program in high school with an emphasis on science and math, and at least three to four years of college-level predental education. Four-fifths of students entering dental school have already earned a bachelor's or master's degree. All dental schools approved by the American Dental Association require applicants to pass a Dental Admission Test (usually one year before they anticipate entering dental school), which measures a student's ability to succeed in dental school. Professional training in a dental school generally requires four academic years. Many dental schools offer an interdisciplinary curriculum, mixing dental students with medical, pharmacy, and other healthcare-profession students.

Clinical training frequently begins in the second year. Most schools located in or near big cities include a department of community dentistry involving the study of sociology, urban ghetto problems, and the treatment of patients from the community. Upon graduation from one of the 60 or so approved dental schools in this country, students are awarded the degree of doctor of dental surgery (D.D.S.) or doctor of dental medicine (D.D.M. or D.M.D.). They must then pass a state board examination, or in some states, the National Board of Dental Examiner's exam. In 16 states and the District of Columbia, a specialist must pass a special state exam in order to be licensed. Generally, dentists licensed in one state are required to take another exam in order to be licensed. Twenty states grant reciprocity to dentists from other states, with appropriate credentials.

Students who wish to specialize (see pages 63–66) must complete postgraduate study of an additional two to four years. A specialist becomes certified only by passing specialty board exams. Dental interns or residents can receive further training in approved hospitals. Once a dentist has graduated from an approved dental school and passed a state licensing exam, the next step is private practice. There are many options: 1) opening one's own office, 2) buying an established practice, 3) joining an existing dentist group, 4) enlisting in the armed services as a commissioned officer, and 5) entering the U.S. Public Health Service, through civil service. Possible settings other than a dental office are hospitals, laboratories, clinics, and schools. Some experienced dentists teach dentistry later in their careers.

Dental Career Checklist

The American Association of Dental Schools offers the following advice for high school students interested in a dentistry career:

- Contact several dental schools and inquire about their specific requirements.
  Talk with admissions officers.

- Enroll in college preparatory classes in chemistry, biology, physics, and math.
- Talk with a counselor or advisor who is knowledgeable about the health professions. Visit that counselor or advisor regularly.
- Talk to your dentist. Ask to spend a day or two in his or her office. The local dental society may be able to direct you to other sources of information.

PRINCIPAL DUTIES

General practitioners in one- or two-dentist offices must be proficient in many areas of dentistry. Many beginning dentists keep overhead down by doing the work of dental hygienists, dental assistants, and laboratory technicians as well, until their patient load increases to the point where they can hire additional staff. Good dental practices can expand exponentially through word of mouth. Dentists as skilled in handling people as they are wielding dental tools can usually expect even more business to come their way from the referrals of satisfied patients.

Specifically, dentists maintain their patients' dental health by preventing and repairing tooth-related problems through extraction, filling, cleaning, or replacement. They also straighten teeth, treat diseased gum tissue, perform mouth or jaw surgery, and fit false teeth. Most dentists establish their own hours and ambiance in setting up offices, although from a practical standpoint they generally try to reflect local habits and tastes.

OUTLOOK

Employment for dentists is expected to grow more slowly than the average for all occupations through the year 2005. Job prospects should continue to improve, however, because the demand for dental care is expected to grow substantially during this same period. Improved dental care over the past several decades means, among other things, that more elderly people will have kept their teeth, and so will require much more care than in the past. Also, improved health insurance plans will permit more people to enjoy good dental healthcare. Finally, because dental school enrollments are down, the competition for employment will be less than would have been expected—meaning better opportunities for younger practitioners.

EARNINGS

The net median income for dentists in private practice is just about $100,000, according to the American Dental Association. For those in specialty practices (see page 63), this figure is about $132,500 annually. Dentists just starting out, of course, will earn less. Because so many dentists are self-employed, they must run their practices like small businesses. As such, they must set their own fees, as well as provide their own retirement benefits, health insurance, and life insurance.

ANOTHER WAY TO GET THERE

The year was 1977, and everything was going George Hetson's way. At age twenty-seven he was so successful in his career as a paint chemist that he'd been offered a partnership in a multimillion dollar start-up company. But Hetson turned the offer down. In his own words:

I didn't have a concrete vision at the time of what I was for, but I knew specifically what I was against. Here's how that went: To keep shipping costs competitive, paint companies must locate their manufacturing facilities inside big cities, where most of the customers are. The plants usually are built in run-down, dangerous neighborhoods, where crime isn't just an item on the six-o'clock news—it's something you confront personally. After a couple of scary experiences, I realized that being a paint chemist meant having to carry a gun to survive. This was a fact of life. I was unhappy with the situation, but at the time I did nothing about it.

Then one day I was on the golf course with a buddy who's a dentist. He knew my feelings about city life, and said: "George, you ought to get out of that rat race and become a dentist." I said "Yeah, yeah." But he pressed the point. "Talk with this friend of mine. She's a college program advisor."

That conversation went well. I'd always had a talent for science. Before I became a paint chemist I was going to be a physicist, so the idea of a career in dentistry didn't seem too far afield.

To make a long story short, I applied to three dental schools and chose Tufts, my former college. I was thirty-one when I graduated, and I interned for a year at a hospital clinic in one of the roughest areas of Brooklyn. This gave me a range of dental experiences I never would have had in ordinary practice. It also made me realize more than ever how much I disliked big-city life.

Even so, for my first practice I rented a chair from a midtown Manhattan dentist, and commuted to an apartment in New Jersey. Why did I do it? I guess I still hadn't committed to total change.

But then, driving home at the end of my tenth day of work, I found myself crawling up a traffic-jammed ramp to the George Washington Bridge. As I sat there, ears ringing from blaring car horns and breathing those choking exhaust fumes, it hit me. I made a U-turn out of there, drove back to my office, terminated my lease, and left. For good.

"Where are we going?" my wife asked when I got home, and I had to admit I didn't know. But within a couple of weeks I found a small practice for sale in a Connecticut town I'd never heard of. I drove up there, looked around, and liked what I saw. The price was right, too.

One thing I wondered about was finding a good golf course. I asked the seller, "How far is it to . . ."

"Thirty to forty minutes," he said before I could finish.

"How did you know what I was going to say?"

"It doesn't matter," the departing dentist said. "Whatever place you name, the answer is thirty to forty minutes."

Which I translated as meaning, this was *really* the country!

That was a magic moment for me. I realized then that the most important thing to me was not money, not a big career, and not even dentistry, per se—but a full, rich quality of life. That was the one thing that, for me, would define true success.

And that's the way it has worked out. By our definition, we truly have it all.

DENTAL SPECIALTIES

Endodontist

Endodontists diagnose and treat diseases and injuries of the dental pulp and other dental tissues that affect the teeth. The pulp is the central portion of the tooth containing nerves and blood vessels. Dead or diseased pulp can be removed by root canal treatment, and replaced with special filling material. Such treatment saves many teeth that would otherwise have to be extracted.

Oral-Maxillofacial Surgeon

Oral-maxillofacial surgeons provide a broad range of diagnostic and treatment services for diseases, injuries, and defects in the head, neck, face, jaws, and associated structures. They also remove some impacted, or heavily wedged third molars (also called wisdom teeth) too difficult to deal with in a regular dental office. Some oral surgeons correct cosmetic problems of the jaws and face, using methods similar to plastic surgery.

ANOTHER WAY TO GET THERE

After graduating magna cum laude from the Harvard School of Dental Medicine in 1982, Dr. David Altobelli completed a residency in oral and maxillofacial surgery at Massachusetts General Hospital. In addition to his private practice, Dr. Altobelli is director of the facial engineering laboratory at Harvard, and an assistant professor at Brigham and Women's Hospital in Boston. His recent focus has been on three-dimensional imaging and computer-assisted analysis for craniofacial surgical planning. The following story was adapted, with permission, from Rensselaer, the Alumni Magazine. *Dr. Altobelli is a graduate of Rensselaer Polytechnic Institute.*

A craniofacial surgical team studies CAT scans of a six-week-old girl. The left side of her face is perfect, but the right side reveals a condition medical experts call a facial cleft. Her blue eye rolls in the middle of her cheek. A fold in her skin runs from the eye to her small, misshapen mouth.

Dr. David Altobelli, after consulting with the team, believes he can redesign the right side of the little girl's face by using her left side as a template. They will use computer modeling to visualize the nature of her problem, as well as a way to solve it when they operate in a few weeks.

"We have a powerful tool for presurgical planning because we can interactively measure, dissect, and manipulate the 3-D models," says Altobelli. "Much of this started after I met a group of GE [General Electric] engineers using 3-D computer images to improve industrial inspection techniques. We quickly moved from their application to a computer visualization of the human body. Since then, we've probably used the technique to plan surgery for more than 20 patients. We call it our 'electric scalpel'."

The breakthrough technology comes from software using data from CAT scans and MRI (magnetic resonance imaging) scans to create three-dimensional computer models of craniofacial anatomy. These new 3-D images, unlike previous models, show soft tissue, such as eyes and skin, as well as bone.

The computer program that made the electronic scalpel possible was written by William Lorensen, a GE computer graphics engineer. Lorensen, a Rensselaer graduate who holds ten patents on his complex software concepts, has worked closely with Altobelli on a number of operations.

"We can get 3-D coordinates that serve as guides to reposition facial features," says Altobelli. "In a couple of cases we've been able to simulate the entire surgery on the computer. That's the edge of the envelope.

"The research is tedious, though. And then there's the constant search for funding. We do some dramatic things for children with malformations, but it's not seen as a big public health problem—which makes the money difficult to come by."

Altobelli's research got started in 1988 with a $60,000 grant from the Foundation for Faces of Children, an organization founded by parents of children with facial deformities. From that came Altobelli's first work station.

But back to the immediate problem. Altobelli and the craniofacial team have decided that the tiny girl with the facial cleft will need two-staged surgery. During the first operation they will insert balloon devices under her skin. These will be inflated gradually to stretch the skin and thereby cover the facial bones when they are repositioned during the second surgery.

No one knows whether the surgery will be successful, or if the little girl's bones will grow as expected. But by continuing to push the envelope, Dr. Altobelli and his fellow surgical and technological pioneers keep that likelihood alive.

(See Chapter 10, Pursuing Careers in Laboratory Medicine and Biomedical Engineering, for another perspective of maxillofacial surgery.)

Oral Pathologist

Oral pathologists study and research the causes, processes, and effects of diseases of the mouth, using laboratory procedures. Some oral pathologists also specialize in forensic dentistry, which applies oral pathology to legal cases. These specialists are frequently called upon to identify corpses by comparing dental records with the teeth and tissues of the deceased. They also provide various kinds of diagnostic and consultative services.

Orthodontist

Orthodontists treat problems related to crooked teeth, missing teeth, and other abnormalities to establish normal function and appearance. These irregularities usually occur as the teeth grow during early childhood. Often the teeth are crowded in the amount of jaw space available, causing an over- or underbite called a malocclusion. Orthodontists correct malocclusions with braces or other mechanical devices that move the teeth into a better position, or by extracting teeth to create more space. They may also use techniques to correct facial structural irregularities.

Pediatric Dentist

Pediatric dentists, also called pedodontists, specialize in treating children from birth through adolescence. They may also, in certain circumstances, treat physically or mentally handicapped patients beyond the age of adolescence.

Periodontist

Periodontists diagnose and treat diseases of the gums and bone supporting the teeth, as well as the ligaments between gums and teeth. Periodontal diseases are responsible for more tooth loss in adults than any other dental problem. Most such problems can be prevented by proper home dental care.

Prosthodontist

Prosthodontists replace missing natural teeth with fixed or removable substitutes such as dentures, bridges, and implants. Sometimes missing teeth are replaced by bridgework cemented to the remaining teeth. Replacements are made of plastic, porcelain, gold or other metals, or combinations of these materials.

Public Health Dentist

Public health dentists specialize in preventing and controlling dental diseases and promoting dental health through organized community efforts.

> Resources: **Department of Career Guidance**
> **American Dental Association**
> **211 E. Chicago Avenue**
> **Chicago, IL 60611**
> **(career information)**
>
> **American Association of Dental Schools**
> **1625 Massachusetts Avenue, NW**
> **Washington, DC 20036**
> **(educational information)**

Dental Vignettes Through History

- In the Middle Ages, dentistry was frequently practiced by jewelers, barbers, and blacksmiths.
- The world's first dental school was founded in Baltimore in 1840 by two American dentists.
- The teeth of the American colonists of the 1600s and 1700s were considered the worst in the world. Poor diet and inadequate cleaning and maintenance caused many colonists to lose at least half their teeth before the age of twenty.
- Since the 1950s, the addition of fluorides to drinking water and toothpastes has greatly reduced tooth decay.

DENTAL HYGIENIST

Preventive dentistry was born in Bridgeport, Connecticut, in 1913, when Dr. Alfred Fones started the first school of dental hygiene. Thirty-four women enrolled in Dr. Fones's first class, many of them doctors' and dentists' wives. They wore long, white starched dresses, boiled dental instruments in huge cauldrons of water as instructed, and pushed foot pedals to activate the tooth polishing machines. What Dr. Fones taught his first class more than 80 years ago essentially holds true today, even though technology has streamlined methodology: The healthiest teeth and those that last the longest belong to the people who clean them thoroughly and often.

PREREQUISITES

Dental hygienists need much of the manual dexterity and self-confidence their dentist employers possess. They are responsible for counseling patients about good preventive dental habits, and so must work well with people. They are expected to know complex procedures well enough to anticipate the dentist's needs, and to work as effective team members.

PREPARATION

Dental hygienists must be licensed by the state in which they practice. They require a minimum of two years of college education, and graduate with a certificate, diploma, or associate's degree. Some programs are longer, with graduates receiving a bachelor's degree. Because the dental hygiene program emphasizes dental and basic science, high school preparation should include courses in biology and chemistry.

PRINCIPAL DUTIES

Because each state has its own regulations regarding dental hygienist responsibilities, the range of duties varies from state to state. Some include screening patients and taking health histories, dental charting, taking and recording blood pressure, exposing and developing x-rays, cleaning teeth, and teaching patients appropriate dental hygiene and nutrition.

OUTLOOK

About 127,000 dental hygienists work in the United States today. Approximately 70 percent of general dentists employ at least one dental hygienist; 30 percent employ two or more. Employment of dental hygienists is expected to grow much faster than the average for all occupations through the year 2005. Older dentists, less likely to hire dental hygienists than recent graduates, will be leaving the profession in increasing numbers over the next several years, thus opening up the profession. As of 1994, dental hygienists had been working at their current jobs for an average of 5.5 years, making this an extremely stable occupation.

EARNINGS

Dental hygienists working 32-hour-or-longer weeks earn an average of $675 weekly, according to the American Dental Association. The average hourly earnings are about $21.00. Part-time hygienists (working without benefits) averaged $22.30 per hour. Benefits usually are dependent on full-time employment, with those working for school systems, public health agencies, and state and federal agencies assured of substantial benefits.

Resource: Division of Professional Development
American Dental Hygienists' Association
444 N. Michigan Avenue, Suite 3400
Chicago, IL 60611
(career and educational information)

DENTAL LABORATORY TECHNICIAN

PREREQUISITES

Because the public rarely sees them, dental laboratory technicians are probably the least known of dental professionals. There are broad areas of specialization available to them, including full and partial dentures, crowns and bridges, ceramics, and orthodontics. Good dental laboratory technicians combine the patience and dexterity of a skilled craft worker with a generous amount of artistic talent. They must be able to execute exacting instructions from the dentist, because each dental fixture must be constructed to precise individual designs.

PREPARATION

Many dental lab technicians are trained on the job; training is also available through community and junior colleges, vocational-technical institutes, and the armed forces. Thirty-seven programs in dental laboratory technology are currently accredited by the Commission on Dental Accreditation, in conjunction with the American Dental Association. These programs provide classroom instruction in dental materials science, oral anatomy, fabrication procedures, ethics, and related subjects.

PRINCIPAL DUTIES

Technicians receive from the dentist a mold, or impression, of the patient's mouth or teeth. They create a model of the patient's mouth by pouring plaster into the impression and allowing it to set. They place the model on an apparatus that traces the bite and movement of the patient's jaw. The technicians then examine the model carefully in relation to adjacent teeth and parts of the mouth, and construct a wax model from which the metal framework for the prosthetic device is made. Once the wax model is complete, technicians pour the cast and form the metal. They then apply porcelain in layers to reach the precise shape and color of the tooth or teeth. The porcelain is baked, and then adjusted and ground to achieve a sealed finish. The final product is an exact replica of the original.

OUTLOOK

Nearly 50,000 dental laboratory technicians work in U.S. commercial dental laboratories, which employ an average of three to five technicians. Some dentists also employ technicians in their private dental offices. Job opportunities probably will remain static until the year 2005. Experienced technicians who have built up favorable reputations with dentists should have good opportunities for establishing laboratories of their own. This in turn will create some additional positions.

EARNINGS

The starting salary of a dental lab technician is approximately $20,000, and varies depending on responsibilities and geographical area. The average annual wage for all dental laboratory workers is about $23,000.

>Resource: **National Association of Dental Laboratories**
>**555 E. Braddock Road**
>**Alexandria, VA 22314**
>**(career and accreditation information)**

For career information about dental assistants, see Chapter 18, Jobs Available to High School Grads.

CHAPTER 7

Pursuing Careers in Dietetics

This is a time in U.S. history when health, nutrition, and fitness have become an integral part of people's lives. Billions of dollars are spent annually on food supplements and weight-loss programs, when minimal attention to sound dietetic principles—plus a sprinkling of prudence—would easily tip the scales back toward healthy diets. (This conclusion in no way applies to people suffering from chronic eating disorders of various kinds, which are discussed in Chapter 11, Pursuing Careers in Mental Health.)

DIETITIAN

Dietitians plan nutrition programs and supervise the preparation and serving of meals with proper nutritional value. They help prevent and treat illnesses by promoting healthy eating habits, and by evaluating clients' diets and suggesting modifications—such as less salt for those with high blood pressure, or reduced fat and sugar for the overweight. They may also be directly responsible for food preparation, requiring the supervision of chefs and other food-service employees.

Dietitians run food-service systems for hospitals, schools, and corporations, and promote sound eating habits through education and research. Major areas of practice are clinical, community, and administrative dietetics. Dietitians also work as educators and researchers.

PREREQUISITES

Because a dietitian's work will vary with the area of specialization, desirable skill sets will vary as well. Anyone interested in the field should try a part-time or summer job with a food company, in a hospital kitchen, or in a restaurant. Seeing dietitians in action, talking with them, and learning as much as possible about the profession are good ways to decide whether to investigate further.

PREPARATION

Those interested in becoming dietitians can get there two ways:

1) ***By enrolling in a Coordinated Program leading to a bachelor's or master's degree.*** *This program combines classroom and supervised practical experience and is accredited by the Commission on Accreditation/Approval for Dietetics Education of the American Dietetic Association (CAADE). Graduates are eligible to take the registration examination for dietitians to become credentialed as an RD, registered dietitian.*

2) ***By enrolling in a Didactic Program in Dietetics,*** *an academic program providing a bachelor's degree that is approved by CAADE. After receiving a degree, graduates then require supervised practical experience by completing either (1) an Approved Preprofessional Practice Program (AP4) or (2) an accredited Dietetic Internship. Upon completion, graduates are eligible to take the exam leading to RD credentialing. Write to The American Dietetics Association (address at end of section) for The Directory of Dietetics Programs, which includes complete listings of CAADE-accredited/approved dietetics education and practice programs.*

PRINCIPAL DUTIES

Dietitians' duties depend on the area of practice they decide to specialize in.

Business dietitians work in food and nutrition-related industries. Areas of interest include product development, sales, marketing, advertising, public relations, purchasing, and many other capacities that satisfy consumers' growing interest in nutrition.

Clinical dietitians are a vital part of the medical team in hospitals, nursing homes, health maintenance organizations, and other healthcare facilities. They work with doctors, nurses, and therapists to help speed patients' recovery and lay the groundwork for long-term health through nutrition. Opportunities for advancement are available by choosing a particular area of nutrition, such as diabetes, cardiology, or pediatrics.

Community dietitians work in public and home health agencies, day-care centers, health and recreation clubs, and in government-funded programs that feed and counsel families, the elderly, pregnant women, children, and the disabled or underprivileged. They also teach, monitor, and advise in other public settings where proper nutrition can help improve quality of life.

Consultant dietitians work part- or full-time, usually under contract with a healthcare facility or in their own private practice. Consultant dietitians in private practice perform nutrition screening and assessment of their own clients and those referred to them by physicians. They offer advice on weight loss, cholesterol reduction, and a variety of other diet-related concerns. Those under contract with healthcare facilities often consult with food service managers, providing expertise on sanitation and safety procedures, budgeting, and portion control. Other clients include athletes, company employees, and nursing home residents.

Educator dietitians work in colleges, universities, and community or technical schools, teaching nutrition to future doctors, nurses, dietitians, and dietetic technicians.

Management dietitians work in healthcare institutions, schools, cafeterias, and restaurants. They are responsible for personnel management, menu planning, budgeting, and purchasing. With more and more Americans recognizing the importance of good nutrition, management dietitians increasingly play a key food-service role.

Research dietitians work in government agencies, food and pharmaceutical companies, and in major universities and medical centers. They conduct or direct experiments to answer critical nutrition questions, and find alternative foods or make dietary recommendations for the public.

Dietary Fat Newsbreaks

The amount of butter consumed by Americans declined from 5.4 pounds per person in 1970 to 4.4 pounds in 1990. However, the average consumption of fats and oils increased from 53 pounds in 1970 to 63 pounds in 1990. Consumption of cooking and salad oils increased from 15.4 pounds in 1970 to 24.2 pounds in 1990, while the consumption of lard dropped dramatically.

* * *

Neurobiologists attribute fat craving to the neurotransmitter galanin, while sociologists believe it to be an evolutionary trait. Experts warn people who indulge themselves on fatty foods to avoid second servings.

OUTLOOK

Employment of dietitians is expected to grow faster than the average profession through the year 2005. The American Dietetic Association has more than 67,000 members.

EARNINGS

According to ADA's membership database, in 1995 of those entry-level RDs who have been employed full-time for one to five years after registration, 24 percent report incomes between $35,000 and $45,000, 63 percent between $25,000 and $35,000. Salary levels vary with location, scope of responsibility, and the supply of job applicants.

Resource: The Commission on Accreditation/Approval for Dietetics Education
The American Dietetic Association
216 W. Jackson Boulevard
Chicago, IL 60606

ANOTHER WAY TO GET THERE

For Donna Poe, M.S., R.D., a self-employed dietitian and nutrition consultant in New Ipswich, New Hampshire, specializing in dietetics was a personal as well as a professional decision. Here's how it came about:

As a child I was very overweight. In high school I joined Weight Watchers [a commercial weight loss organization] and was successful in losing weight, but I was left with several unanswered questions that my group leader was unqualified to answer. At about that same time, my guidance counselor asked me what I wanted to do with the rest of my life. Growing up I had an interest in two career fields: healthcare and education. I found nutrition to be a wonderful combination of the two because the field of dietetics is dynamic—it is constantly growing and changing, and the opportunities are endless.

Food habits are very personal. It is rewarding to see that a simple change in one's eating habits can result in a tremendous change in quality of life: more confidence, greater stamina, and a boost in self-esteem. Every May for the past five years, I've received a note and photo from a successful client to celebrate the anniversary of reaching her goal!

I look for creative ways to make nutrition information interesting. I use visuals to portray fat grams in various processed foods—melted Crisco packaged in various amounts, for example—and I have a weight vest (a vest with removable one- to twenty-pound weights), so clients can feel the effect that extra fat pounds have on their cardiovascular system.

One of the greatest challenges for me is to disseminate all the nutrition advice out there—some of it sound, some of it unsubstantiated—and present it to the public in a clear, understandable way. Another challenge is to become "politically savvy" because of the climate regarding healthcare issues today. Several states now have licensure for registered dietitians. New Hampshire does not. What this means is that consumers need to be wary of whom they turn to for nutrition advice. My profession is also working toward insurance coverage for nutrition services. We continue to gather statistics of cost-effectiveness, and it is proven that nutrition therapy saves healthcare dollars.

I am now a self-employed nutrition consultant/registered dietitian and have the pleasure of working in a variety of settings. There's never a dull moment. For example, here are some of my assignments over the past year (the first two are ongoing):

- Counsel individuals on ways to lower their cholesterol
- Lead group weight-management classes
- Addressed a "Nannies' Conference" on "Ways to Jazz up Kids' Nutrition"
- Instructed a group of high school wrestlers on "Gaining the Competitive Edge With Good Nutrition"
- Talked with women at a cancer support group meeting

- Led nutrition-consciousness-raising supermarket tours
- Generated nutrition analysis food labels for a local retail bakery.

My advice to anyone entering the field today is to gain years of practical experience before going it alone. Being self-employed requires confidence that comes with varied exposures to a variety of situations. Also, it's important to have fellow nutrition professionals you can call on to bounce off ideas and get input from different perspectives.

DIETETIC TECHNICIAN

Dietetic technicians work together with registered dietitians in a number of different settings, such as hospitals, public health nutrition programs, and long-term care facilities. They also work in child nutrition and school lunch programs, community wellness centers, health clubs, nutrition programs for the elderly, food companies, restaurants, and food-service management.

PREREQUISITES

An ability to work with people and a strong interest in food and nutrition are qualities a dietetic technician should have. Motivation, the initiative to work independently, and good problem-solving skills are other desirable assets. Computer skills are a plus. Dietetic technicians use computers for everything from inputting inventory and payroll to charting patients' nutritional progress.

PREPARATION

To become a dietetic technician, students must complete a two-year CADADE-approved program leading to an associate degree. The program combines classroom and supervised practical experience. Graduates of the program are eligible to take the Registration Examination leading to credentialing as a Registered Dietetic Technician (DTR).

PRINCIPAL DUTIES

Dietetic technicians' responsibilities are as varied as the settings in which they work. They may screen patients to identify nutrition problems. They often provide patient education and counseling to individuals or groups, develop menus and recipes, supervise food-service personnel, purchase food, and monitor inventory.

OUTLOOK

The employment prospects for dietetic technicians are roughly the same as for dietitians over the next several years.

EARNINGS

According to The American Dietetic Association's 1995 membership database, 23 percent of all registered dietetic technicians employed full-time for one to five years report annual gross incomes of less than $20,000, 62 percent report between $20,000 and $30,000, and 12 percent report incomes between $30,000 and $40,000. Salary levels vary based on location, scope of responsibility, and talent pool.

Resource: **The American Dietary Association**
216 W. Jackson Boulevard
Chicago, IL 60606

CHAPTER 8

Pursuing Careers in Eyecare

More than half of all adults and children in the United States wear eyeglasses or contact lenses. And after the age of forty nearly everyone suffers from presbyopia, a condition usually accompanied by a suspicion that if one's arms were only three inches longer, the morning newspaper's front page stories would snap into focus.

Another million or more Americans suffer from glaucoma, the most dangerous of eye diseases and the leading cause of blindness in this country. Glaucoma occurs in a variety of forms, but it can be treated successfully if diagnosed and treated early. Cataracts—a cloudiness that prevents light rays from striking the retina unimpeded—is the second leading cause of blindess. Diseases associated with other parts of the body can also affect the eyes—diabetes, for example, or high blood pressure.

The upside of these grim facts is that a whole range of professionals are now at work or in training to bring the incidence of eye-related diseases under control. Here are some of them.

OPHTHALMOLOGIST

An ophthalmologist specializes in the treatment of the eyes. After completing medical school and an internship, this doctor goes on for three to five years of specialized training in the medical specialty of ophthalmology. Ophthalmologists can provide complete eyecare. In addition to prescribing glasses and contact lenses, they diagnose and treat eye diseases, treat injuries to the eyes, perform various surgeries, and direct remedial activities to aid in regaining vision or—by instructing patients in eye exercises—to use sight remaining. They treat conditions like glaucoma, cataracts, retinal detachment, and obstruction of tear ducts. They also are trained to identify the symptoms of more generalized problems that may affect the eyes, such as hypertension or diabetes. See Chapter 2, Career Opportunities as Doctors, for additional information on the training, duties, and career outlook for ophthalmologists.

Resource: American Academy of Ophthalmology
655 Beach Street
San Francisco, CA 94120

OPTOMETRIST

Doctors of optometry examine people's eyes to diagnose vision problems and eye disease. In most states they are licensed as well to treat such eye diseases as conjunctivitis and corneal infections, and to prescribe appropriate medication. Optometrists use instruments and observation to examine eye health and to test patients' visual acuity, depth and color perception, and ability to focus and coordinate the eyes. Unlike ophthalmologists, optometrists are not trained to perform eye surgery or treat all diseases. When they diagnose conditions that require care beyond their scope of practice, they refer patients to other practitioners, usually ophthalmologists.

PREREQUISITES

Business ability, self-discipline, and the ability to deal tactfully with patients are essential for success. Because most optometrists are self-employed, they also handle the business aspects of running an office, such as hiring employees, keeping records, and ordering equipment and supplies. Optometrists who operate franchise optical stores may also have some of these duties. A growing number of optometrists are in partnership or group practice. Others work as salaried employees of ophthalmologists, in hospitals, or for HMOs.

PREPARATION

All states require that optometrists be licensed. Applicants for license must have a Doctor of Optometry degree from an accredited optometry school and pass both a written and a clinical state board examination. The four-year optometry school program is preceded by at least three years of preoptometric study at an accredited college or university. (Most optometry students have a bachelor's degree.) Seventeen U.S. schools of optometry are accredited by the Council on Optometric Education of the American Optometric Association.

PRINCIPAL DUTIES

Other than those duties mentioned above, optometrists sometimes specialize in work with children, the elderly, or partially sighted people who use specialized visual aids. Others develop ways to protect workers' eyes from on-the-job strain and injury. Some specialize in contact lenses, sports vision, or vision therapy.

OUTLOOK

Employment for optometrists is expected to grow at roughly the same pace as the average for all occupations through the year 2005. The vast majority of Americans over the age of forty-five visit optometrists or ophthalmologists because of a virtually universal onset of vision problems in middle age.

EARNINGS

Optometrists just out of school earn an average of $45,000 during their first year of practice. Overall, the median annual net income for experienced optometrists is about $80,000. Optometrists in business for themselves tend to earn more than salaried optometrists.

    Resource: **American Optometric Association**
                                 Educational Services
                                 243 North Lindbergh Boulevard
                                 St. Louis, MO 63141

Brain Injury and Optometry

Several months after a terrible motorcycle accident left him with blurred eyesight, chronic dizziness, and an uncontrollable shaking of the head, David Tela was understandably despondent. Tela's psychologist suspected traumatic brain injury. But when he referred the young man to an optometrist, of all things, Tela was incredulous.

He was even more incredulous when, 30 minutes after meeting Dr. William Padula, a Guilford, Connecticut optometrist, he put down his cane and walked perfectly without it. "It was amazing," said Tela. "For the first time I could stand straight. My eyes filled with tears. I could hardly believe it."

What Dr. Padula had observed, after listening carefully to Tela's account of the accident, was "midline shift." Tela's brain believed that the midpoint of his body was far off-center. Consequently, he felt continuously off-balance and was unable to walk without a cane.

Padula, a world-renowned expert for his work with traumatic brain injury, gave Tela a pair of prism lenses, which helped the patient's brain realign its impression.

Three years later Tela still cannot believe the difference. "I still wear the prism glasses, but at a much weaker strength now."

OPHTHALMIC MEDICAL TECHNICIAN/TECHNOLOGIST

Ophthalmic medical technicians and technologists are qualified by academic and clinical training to perform ophthalmic procedures under the supervision of an ophthalmologist. (An additional category, "ophthalmic medical assistant," is no longer sanctioned by the Commission on Accreditation of Allied Health Education Programs.)

PREREQUISITES

Ophthalmic medical technologists perform all duties performed by technicians, but they are expected to do so at a higher level of expertise and to exercise considerable technical clinical judgment.

PREPARATION

Programs are generally one year long for technicians, and two years for technologists. Applicants are required to have a high school diploma or equivalent. The curriculum includes courses in anatomy and physiology, medical terminology, medical laws and ethics, psychology, ocular anatomy and physiology, ophthalmic optics, microbiology, and diseases of the eye.

PRINCIPAL DUTIES

Ophthalmic medical technicians and technologists render supportive services to the ophthalmologist. They are employed primarily by ophthalmologists but may be employed by medical institutions, clinics, or physician groups specializing in ophthalmology. They may be involved with patients of an ophthalmologist in any setting for which the ophthalmologist is responsible.

OUTLOOK

Opportunities for ophthalmic technicians and technologists are favorable, particularly in practices that involve more than the ophthalmologist.

EARNINGS

Entry-level salaries for technicians and technologists average about $24,000—a little above for technologists, whose preparation has been more rigorous; a little below for technicians.

Resource: Joint Review Committee for Ophthalmic Medical Personnel
            2025 Woodlane Drive
            St. Paul, MN 55125

Headaches and Vision Problems

Daniel Rallison, of Wise Eyes Optical Inhouse Service, in St. Albert, Ontario, lists seven separate vision-associated problems that can lead to headaches.

- Poor eyesight: The brain works harder to clarify the image, which takes more concentration and mental pressure.
- Light source: Constant use of a computer screen or working in a bright light can lead to excessive strain on the eyes.
- Distortions: Imperfections in inexpensive sunglasses or drugstore reading glasses may cause distortions leading to headaches.
- Progressive bifocals: Progressive bifocals (without the lines) have a reading power that changes gradually from the top of the lens to the bottom. The "blur zone" can cause headache problems.
- Body position: Bifocal users must raise their chins to use the reading portion of the lens. This can result in neck misalignment and subsequent headaches.

- External pressure: Improperly fitted frames can cause pressure points near the eyes or cheekbones that can in turn cause headaches.
- Exhaustion: Working at computer screens for prolonged periods can tire the eyes, causing strain leading to headaches.
- Glare: Glare is reflected light from a flat surface, seen as a white spot. Over time, the spot will strain the eyes and cause headaches.

OPTICIAN

Opticians, also called dispensing opticians, fit eyeglasses and contact lenses, following prescriptions written by ophthalmologists or optometrists.

PREREQUISITES

Because opticians deal directly with the public, they should be tactful and pleasant and communicate well. A knowledge of physics, basic anatomy, algebra, geometry, and mechanical drawing is valuable because training usually includes instruction in optical applications of these subjects.

PREPARATION

Some employers hire people with no background in opticianry, or those who have worked as ophthalmic laboratory technicians (see page 81). Training may be informal, on-the-job, or formal apprenticeship. Others seek people with college level training in opticianry. In the 21 states that license dispensing opticians, those without formal college-level education train from two to four years as apprentices. Some states that license dispensing opticians allow graduates to take the licensure exam immediately upon graduation. Others require a few months to one year of experience.

PRINCIPAL DUTIES

Opticians examine written prescriptions to determine lens specifications. They recommend eyeglass frames, lenses, and lens coatings based on the prescription and the customer's occupation, habits, and facial features. Opticians also fix, adjust, and refit broken frames, and instruct clients about eyeglass wear and care. They keep records on customer prescriptions, work orders, and payments; track inventory and sales; and perform other administrative duties.

OUTLOOK

About 63,000 men and women work as opticians in the United States. Employment is expected to increase faster than the average for all occupations through the year 2005.

EARNINGS

Salaries for opticians in retail stores average about $26,700. The beginning average salary for licensed and certified opticians is a little under $21,000. Those who have been in the field for ten years or more average almost $30,000.

    Resources: **Opticians Association of America**
                        10341 Democracy Lane
                        Fairfax, VA 22030

                        Commission on Opticianry Accreditation
                        10111 Martin Luther King, Jr. Highway, Suite 100
                        Bowie, MD 20720

OPHTHALMIC LABORATORY TECHNICIAN

Ophthalmic laboratory technicians make prescription eyeglass lenses. Some manufacture lenses for other optical instuments, such as telescopes and binoculars.

PREREQUISITES

Manual dexterity and the ability to do precision work is essential.

PREPARATION

Most employers prefer high school graduates. Those who have had courses in science and mathematics are even more desirable. Nearly all ophthalmic laboratory technicians learn their skills on the job. Some attend one of the programs in optical technology offered by vocational-technical colleges or trade schools.

PRINCIPAL DUTIES

Prescription lenses are curved in such a way that light is focused correctly onto the retina (the back of the eye), thus improving vision. Ophthalmic laboratory technicians cut, grind, edge, and finish lenses according to specifications provided by ophthalmologists, optometrists, or opticians, and then assemble the lenses with frames to produce finished glasses. They start on simple tasks such as marking or blocking lenses for grinding, then progress to lens-grinding, lens-cutting, and eyeglass assembly.

OUTLOOK

About 19,000 men and women hold jobs as ophthalmic laboratory technicians. The expectation is that jobs in this field will increase about as fast as the average for all occupations between now and the year 2005.

EARNINGS

The beginning average salary for ophthalmic laboratory technicians is a little over $15,000. Those with ten years or more experience average just under $25,000.

>Resource: Commission on Opticianry Accreditation
>10111 Martin Luther King, Jr. Highway, Suite 100
>Bowie, MD 20720

Following are three other optometric support positions you may be interested in learning more about.

A *paraoptometric* works under the direct supervision of a licensed doctor of optometry, collects patient data, administers routine yet technical tests of the patient's visual capabilities, and assists in office management. The paraoptometric may assist the optometrist in providing primary patient care examination and treatment services, including contact lenses, low vision, vision therapy, optical dispensing, and office management. State laws may limit, restrict, or otherwise affect the duties that may be performed by the paraoptometric.

An *optometric assistant* is a paraoptometric primarily involved in front office procedures, optical dispensing, and contact lens patient-education. The optometric assistant may be trained on the job or may have completed a formal education program of less than one academic year, and succesfully completed the National Optometric Assistant Registry Examination.

An *optometric technician* is a paraoptometric who is prepared for widely diversified duties through academic and clinical experience. Technicians work directly with optometrists in the areas of patient examination and treatment, including contact lenses, low-vision correction, vision therapy, optical dispensing, and office management. The optometric technician may have completed a college program in optometric technology of a minimum of one academic year, or qualify for the position by successfully completing the Optometric Technician Registry Examination.

>Resource: American Optometric Association
>243 N. Lindbergh Boulevard
>St. Louis, MO 63141
>(career and education information)

CHAPTER 9

Pursuing Careers in Health Information Management

Just a few decades ago most hospitals in the United States maintained central libraries of patient records, kept in good order by medical record librarians. Two relatively recent influences, however, transformed "medical record keeping" into "health information management." One was the computerization of many more medical records (for a growing, longer-living population) than ever before. The other was an increased need to accommodate two divergent constitutional principles: privacy and freedom of information.

Health information management (HIM) professionals still collect, analyze, and store information. Their objectives today, though, have become vastly more complex. Hospitals, clinics, and other healthcare entities must be aware of such tangential issues as:
- Allowing access to patient data by only those directly involved in the patient's care
- Reviewing security systems on a regular basis
- Recording and storing files in protected areas with controlled access
- Keeping records of unauthorized attempts to obtain patient information

The reason for this level of confidentiality protection is that health information can be used against individuals. Insurance companies, for example, may use patient medical data as a basis for making underwriting decisions. Politicians have had elections and careers destroyed because of public disclosure of past mental health treatment.

Still, the basic function of HIM professionals is to manage hundreds of millions of computerized and paper health records. Essentially, these professionals are responsible for:
- Collecting data from a variety of sources
- Monitoring the integrity of the data
- Ensuring appropriate access to the data
- Protecting the confidentiality of the data
- Managing the analysis, interpretation, and use of the data

Although many HIM professionals work in hospitals and clinics, many others are employed in physicians' offices, private insurance companies, law firms, mental health facilities, nursing homes, consulting firms, and software companies.

A variety of occupations and career paths are available to those interested in the HIM field, most of which lead to certification in one of three basic occupations: (1) medical record administrator; (2) medical record technician; and (3) coding specialist. A fourth HIM occupation, medical transcriptionist, is administered by a separate professional association and is described beginning on page 88.

PREREQUISITES

Success in all four of these areas depends on an affinity for working with data (to a greater extent, that is, than working with people or "things"). Because accuracy is essential, the most crucial characteristics are an ability to concentrate and to pay close attention to detail. Frequent deadlines also require people who are unflappable under pressure. Doctors, nurses, and the rest of the healthcare team respect the information management specialist as the expert in medical data.

Medical record administrators and technicians whose objectives include promotion to management need to prepare themselves for this increased responsibility and the requisite supervisory roles that accompany it. Those of you in this position should consider taking management courses, as well as consulting a boss you respect and feel comfortable with. Managerial HIM positions require an ability to hire, train, and coach people; anticipate and solve problems; delegate responsibility; work within a budget and keep to a schedule; and plan for future projects and activities.

MEDICAL RECORD ADMINISTRATOR

PREPARATION

To become a medical record administrator (MRA), a high school graduate must earn a bachelor's degree from one of the 170 accredited medical record administration college or university programs. Courses in most programs include anatomy, physiology, biology, medical terminology and diseases, legal aspects of medical records, coding and abstraction of data, statistics, data bases, and basic computer software courses. Upon graduation, individuals are eligible to take a national registration examination offered every October by the American Health Information Management Association. Those passing this examination become registered record administrators (RRA), with access to considerably greater career opportunity than those without this credential.

If you already have a college degree, you can earn a postgraduate certificate in health information management, or take the independent study program to attain sufficient credentials.

The American Health Information Management Association's Foundation of Record Education (FORE) offers scholarships and loans to health information management students.

PRINCIPAL DUTIES

A registered record administrator interacts with other members of medical, financial, and administrative staffs to ensure accurate, up-to-the-minute data, as well as overall protection of the information system. RRAs who are also departmental managers frequently determine health information policies, budgets, and resources; act as liaison with other departments; evaluate employee performance; educate the medical staff and ancillary departments to assure quality information; and serve on policy-making committees such as quality assurance and utilization review.

The health information systems set up by RRAs must meet medical, administrative, ethical, and legal requirements. Professionals in record administration plan and develop medical record systems, as well as institutional data. They are in charge of these records and responsible for the release of any information they contain.

OUTLOOK

Careers in health information management in general and medical record administration in particular are rapidly expanding. Additional occupations created within the past several years include quality assurance manager, risk manager, HIM home health coordinator, and HIM long-term care director. According to an American Hospital Association study, by the year 2000 the number of unfilled jobs for RRAs will have increased by 54 percent.

EARNINGS

Medical record administrator salaries vary by location, experience, and whether certified or not. Entry-level administrators earn from $17,000 to $21,000 annually. With additional education, experience, and certification, RRAs earn between $22,400 and $31,000. With an advanced degree the salary can go to $40,000 and above. Promotions to advanced managerial positions demand higher salaries. Here are the ranges for three representative positions:

Health Information Department Director: $30,000–$80,000
HIM Department Assistant Director: $25,000–$65,000
HIM Consultant: $25,000–$100,000

MEDICAL RECORD TECHNICIAN

PREPARATION

Medical record technicians (MRTs) perform a variety of technical health information functions, including organizing, analyzing, and evaluating health information; compiling various administrative and health statistics; and coding diseases, operations, procedures, and other therapies.

High school graduates can become MRTs by completing a two-year associate's program from an accredited medical record technology college or university program, or by passing an independent study program in medical record technology offered by the American Health Information Management Association (AHIMA). Graduates from accredited MRT programs are eligible to take the national registration exam administered by AHIMA. Successful candidates are certified as accredited record technicians (ARTs), and can use the ART credential after their names. ARTs have much greater career advancement and earnings leverage than do MRTs.

The AHIMA independent study program is an alternative to traditional classroom settings, an aid for those with day jobs who need their regular paychecks. Those successfully completing the program can take the national certification exam to become an ART. Before enrolling in an AHIMA independent study, students must complete a college-level English composition course, as well as at least one of the following college courses: math, human anatomy and physiology, or introduction to computers. Tuition for a management record technician independent study course is $2,000, including registration.

PRINCIPAL DUTIES

Most medical record technicians assist medical record administrators. MRTs maintain and use a variety of health information indexes; they create special registries and storage and retrieval systems; input and retrieve computerized health data; supervise health information staff such as medical record clerks, coding specialists, and medical record transcriptionists; and control the use and release of health information.

OUTLOOK

According to the American Hospital Association, employment prospects through the year 2000 are excellent. In a population that is both growing and aging, demand for MRTs will continue to exceed supply. Technicians with two-year associate degrees and ART status will have the best prospects. Although most employment opportunities will continue to be in hospitals, other possibilities are in extended-care facilities, ambulatory-care facilities, health management organizations, medical group practices, and nursing homes.

EARNINGS

Salaries of entry-level medical record technicians average about $17,500 annually. Experienced technicians in supervisory roles can earn between $22,500 and $31,500 per year. Those with a bachelor's degree or who are ART-certified can expect an average annual salary of about $37,000.

Patient Records and Confidentiality

Of a proposal to establish a computer network containing all information on all patients in the United States, Beverly Woodward writes in the November 23, 1995 issue of *The New England Journal of Medicine:*

Patient confidentiality is already threatened as more parties, including insurers, employers, and detectives, claim the right to access medical records. A growing number of employees of healthcare facilities have access to computerized patient records and these people may be paid by outside parties to disclose information. Disclosure of such information can lead to discrimination by businesses, employers, schools, and families.

Some argue that a national medical data network would foster research that could benefit public health, and such benefits are more important than individual privacy. However, the loss of privacy could cause people to not seek care or alter what they say to doctors. Congressional bills that establish a national data network should make provisions to protect patient confidentiality.

CODING SPECIALIST

PREPARATION

Coding is central to both healthcare reimbursement and clinical analysis. As such it requires highly trained and accurate professionals. Coding specialists are called upon to analyze health records and assign and sequence numerical categories to classify medical data. Coding specialists require a high school diploma or equivalent. A coding education can be attained through workshops, seminars, and coding tracks within medical record administration or medical record technology programs. On-the-job coding experience and a solid coding education are needed to take the certification examination to become a certified coding specialist. The American Health Information Management Association also offers an independent study program in coding.

PRINCIPAL DUTIES

The coding specialist applies numerical codes to report diagnoses and procedures for all payers, including the federal government and private insurance companies. These codes are also needed for comparing and tracking diseases, clinical research, statistical reporting, market data, and long-range planning.

OUTLOOK

The outlook for coding specialists is extremely promising, mirroring the prospects for both record administrators and record technicians.

EARNINGS

Entry-level coding specialists can expect an hourly wage of between $6 and $10 per hour.

Salary for experienced certified coding specialists depends on location, size of the organization and whether it is for-profit, not-for-profit, or a governmental institution, in some situations exceeding $20 per hour.

For information on scholarships and loans for health information management students, contact:

Foundation of Record Education
American Health Information Management Association
919 N. Michigan Avenue, Suite 1400
Chicago, IL 60611-1683
(312) 787-2672

MEDICAL TRANSCRIPTIONIST

Medical transcriptionists are medical language specialists who interpret and transcribe dictation by physicians and other healthcare professionals. They transcribe patient assessments, therapeutic procedures, clinical courses, and diagnoses, to name a few. They also edit dictated material for grammar and clarity.

PREREQUISITES

Successful medical transcriptionists excel in English grammar, punctuation, and spelling skills, and have a strong interest in the medical language and a good memory for new terms. They must also have good listening skills, both because many physicians speak English as a second language, and the dictation often occurs in a noisy environment. Transcriptionists must have a knowledge of computers and word-processing software and be able to work for long hours at a computer or word processor, often in a stressful environment.

PREPARATION

Classes for medical transcription can be found in many community colleges and home-study programs. The American Association for Medical Transcription (AAMT) neither offers a self-study program nor evaluates or accredits schools offering such programs. It does, however, provide a checklist of questions to ask school administrators regarding the quality and length of any specific program. Such a program, according to the AAMT, should include classes in English grammar and punctuation, anatomy and physiology, disease processes, beginning and advanced medical terminology, medico-legal and ethical issues, professional development, and transcription technology. By passing written and practical entry-level examinations, experienced transcriptionists attain status as certified medical transcriptionists (CMT). In order to keep this credential, a CMT must take at least 30 continuing education credits every three years.

PRINCIPAL DUTIES

Medical transcriptionists work in hospitals, clinics, physician offices, transcription services, insurance companies, and home healthcare agencies. Some transcriptionists work in their homes as subcontractors or freelancers. The work is largely sedentary, involving continuous use of earphones, keyboard, foot control, and video display terminal.

OUTLOOK

Qualified transcriptionists are in great demand. Entry-level candidates will have a more difficult time. The current heavy workloads in most hospitals and clinics leaves little time or budget for on-the-job training. Graduates who offer to volunteer for a short time, or those willing to start in a lesser position until a vacancy occurs (as a receptionist, for example) will have the best chance.

EARNINGS

Earnings vary widely by geographical area and level of experience. Annual salaries can range from $15,000 to $30,000; and are higher for CMTs.

> **Resource:** **American Association for Medical Transcription**
> **P.O. Box 576187**
> **Modesto, CA 95357**

CHAPTER 10

Pursuing Careers in Laboratory Medicine and Biomedical Engineering

Most of the breakthroughs and innovations in medicine through the years have occurred in the laboratory, where a variety of specialists perform tests to aid in the detection, diagnosis, and treatment of disease.

Another recent area of innovation is in the area of biomedical engineering. An introduction to this important and fast-growing field begins on page 96.

PATHOLOGIST

Medical pathologists study the nature, cause, and development of diseases, as well as the structural and functional changes caused as a result of them. They examine body tissues, fluids, secretions, and other specimens using laboratory technology, and determine a disease's presence and stage of progression. They act as consultants to other medical practitioners. They perform autopsies to determine the cause of death, the nature and extent of a disease, and the effects of treatment. They may direct the activities of pathology departments in medical schools, hospitals, clinics, the medical examiner's office, or a research institute. They may be designated, according to specialty, as clinical pathologists, forensic pathologists, neuropathologists, or surgical pathologists.

Pathologists must meet all of the requirements for licensure as other specialized physicians listed in Chapter 2, Career Opportunities as Doctors. They rank among the top half-dozen most highly compensated physicians by specialty, as listed in the table on page 27.

Resource: American Society for Investigative Pathology
9650 Rockville Pike
Bethesda, MD 20814

PATHOLOGIST ASSISTANT

Pathologist assistants (PAs) are highly trained professionals who provide services in anatomic pathology under the supervision of a pathologist.

PREREQUISITES

Like those who choose careers as physicians' assistants, those interested in a pathologist assistant profession may be unable or unwilling to make a commitment to become a pathologist, whether in terms of time, finances, or academics.

PREPARATION

Four schools currently provide academic and practical training for prospective pathologist assistants, leading to either a bachelor's degree or a master's degree. Wayne State University offers a bachelor's degree; Duke University, Quinnipiac College (Hamden, CT), and the University of Maryland offer master's degrees. (As of the publication date of *Your Career in Healthcare,* the University of Wyoming had initiated a PA program, pending approval of the state legislature.) To qualify for pathologist assistant programs, candidates must have enough biological and chemical sciences to begin the study of pathology (preferably with heavy emphasis on basic sciences such as cell biology and biochemistry.) Some programs require either Graduate Record Examination (GRE) or Medical College Admission Test (MCAT) scores for entry.

PRINCIPAL DUTIES

Routine duties may include description and dissection of surgical tissue; summarization of patient's medical records; performance of post-mortem examinations with subsequent dissection and dictation of data; supervising anatomic laboratory technicians and other lab personnel; teaching residents, medical students, and other allied health professionals; assuming laboratory administrative duties; and managing computer systems. Employment opportunities may be found in medical centers, teaching institutions, private and community hospitals, research laboratories, and commercial reference laboratories.

OUTLOOK

The demand for pathologist assistants is high, because of a shortage nationwide. Over the past five years there have been at least four job opportunities for each graduate.

EARNINGS

Salaries vary with geographic location and type of employing institution. Entry level salaries start at approximately $40,000.

    Resource: American Association of Pathologists' Assistants
                                183 East Main Street, Suite 1200
                                Rochester, NY 14604

HUMAN GENETIC COUNSELOR

In recent years, advances in basic biological knowledge, especially at the genetic level, have spurred the field of biotechnology. The first such program, at the master's degree level, was established at Sarah Lawrence College in 1969. Today there are 20 such programs.

PREREQUISITES

A strong affinity for biological sciences and a high degree of empathy to work with families in stressful times are necessary qualities.

PREPARATION

The human genetic program leads to a master's degree. The required curriculum can be completed on a full-time basis in two years. In the first year, students are placed in clinical settings and in a cytogenetics laboratory. In the second year, students spend all their fieldwork time in supervised rotations at three different genetic counseling clinics. The National Society of Genetic Counselors offers two versions of an "Information and Resource Packet": one for high school students and one for college students or professionals considering a career change. To request the appropriate packet, telephone (610) 872-7608.

PRINCIPAL DUTIES

The genetic counselor helps families incorporate information about familial disorders. Often families must make crucial decisions at times of emotional distress—decisions that will have long-term effects on their lives. Counselors also participate in clinical research projects and teach consumers, general practitioners, nurses, and social workers about genetic disorders.

The Fragile X Syndrome

The Fragile X syndrome is an inherited defect of the X chromosome that causes mental retardation. Fragile X syndrome is the most common cause of mental retardation in males after Down's syndrome.

    The disorder occurs within families according to an X-linked recessive pattern of inheritance. Although males are mainly affected, women are able to carry the genetic defect responsible for the disorder and pass it on to some of their daughters, who in turn become carriers.

Approximately one in 1,500 men is affected by the condition; one in 1,000 women is a carrier. In addition to being retarded, affected males are generally tall, physically strong, and have a prominent nose and jaw. About one third of female carriers show some degree of intellectual impairment.

There is no treatment for the condition. If a woman has a history of the syndrome in her family, it is useful to seek genetic counseling regarding the risk of a child being affected.

OUTLOOK

About 1,400 genetic counselors are at work today, approximately 10 percent of them nurses with graduate training. The employment outlook is expected to be excellent, after a temporary downturn attributed to the employment shakeup in the healthcare industry in general.

EARNINGS

The median average annual salary for a graduate of one of the master's degree programs for those with up to two years of experience is $34,500. The comparable figure for those with 10 to 14 years experience is $47,600. Some experienced practitioners earn $75,000 or more.

Resource: National Society of Genetic Counselors
233 Canterbury Drive
Wallingford, PA 19086

MEDICAL TECHNOLOGIST

Also called clinical laboratory technologists, medical technologists perform laboratory tests in a number of specialty areas essential to the detection, diagnosis, and treatment of disease. They work under the supervision of specialists in the biological sciences.

PREREQUISITES

Clinical laboratory personnel need analytical judgment and the ability to work under pressure. Close attention to detail is essential because small differences or changes in test substances or numerical readouts can be crucial for patient care. Manual dexterity and normal color vision are highly desirable, as are a familiarity with computers and well-developed problem-solving skills.

PREPARATION

Medical technologists generally have a bachelor's degree in medical technology or in one of the life sciences, or a combination of formal training and work experience. Master's degrees in medical technology and related clinical laboratory sciences provide training for specialized areas of laboratory work or teaching, administration, or research.

Bachelor's degree programs in medical technology include courses in chemistry, biological sciences, microbiology, mathematics, and specialized courses devoted to knowledge and skills used in the clinical laboratory. The American Medical Association's Committee on Allied Health Education and Accreditation accredits more than 800 programs providing education for medical technologists and technicians.

PRINCIPAL DUTIES

Technologists in small laboratories perform many types of tests, while those in specialty or large laboratories perform tests within a single specialty. For example:
- *Clinical chemistry technologists* prepare specimens and analyze the chemical and hormonal contents of body fluids.
- *Microbiology technologists* examine and identify bacteria and other microorganisms.
- *Blood bank technologists* collect, type, and prepare blood and its components for transfusions.
- *Immunology technologists* examine elements and responses of the human immune system to foreign bodies.
- *Cytotechnologists,* who have specialized training, prepare slides of body cells and microscopically examine these cells for abnormalities that may signal the beginning of a cancerous growth.

OUTLOOK

The fastest growth for clinical laboratory technologists is expected to be in independent medical laboratories because hospitals send them a greater share of their testing. Advances in laboratory automation and the development of simpler tests (allowing more people to perform them) will slow the growth of jobs in other settings. Overall, employment is expected to grow about as fast as the average for all occupations for the next several years.

EARNINGS

The median annual salary for medical technologists is just over $31,000. (The median for cytotechnologists is about $37,000.) The average minimum is just under $30,000, and the average maximum is about $44,000.

Resources: American Medical Technologists
710 Higgins Road
Park Ridge, IL 60068

American Association of Blood Banks
1117 N. 19th Street, Suite 600
Arlington, VA 22209

American Society of Cytology
1015 Chestnut Street, Suite 1518
Philadelphia, PA 19107

Committee on Allied Health Education and Accreditation
515 N. State Street
Chicago, IL 60610

MEDICAL TECHNICIAN

PREPARATION

Medical laboratory technicians generally have an associate degree from a community or junior college, or a diploma or certificate from a vocational or technical school. A few technicians learn on the job. The National Accrediting Agency for Clinical Laboratory Sciences accredits more than 200 certificate associate degree programs and 40 to 50 certificate programs.

PRINCIPAL DUTIES

Medical laboratory technicians perform routine tests and laboratory procedures. Technicians may prepare specimens and operate automatic analyzers, or they may perform manual tests following detailed instructions. Like technologists, they may work in several areas of the clinical laboratory or specialize in just one.

Histology technicians cut and stain tissue specimens for microscopic examination by pathologists.

Phlebotomists draw and test blood. They usually work under the supervision of medical technologists or laboratory managers.

OUTLOOK

Same as for clinical technologists.

EARNINGS

The median annual salary for laboratory technicians in general is a little less than $25,000; for histology technicians, just over $26,500; for phlebotomists, just under $17,000.

>   Resource: **National Certification Agency for Medical Laboratory Personnel**
>   7910 Woodmont Avenue, Suite 1301
>   Bethesda, MD 20814

The Do-It-Yourself Home Lab

The disposable home test kit is about as portable as a TV remote control and easier to follow than a cake recipe. Drug stores are selling more than $1.5 billion worth of kits. Johnson & Johnson, which markets several types, conducted a survey of 1,000 Americans and found that 84 percent think the kits are more convenient than screenings at a doctor's office or laboratory, and that 60 percent of households have used a home medical test.

Many home test kits are designed to screen for the presence or absence of a specific chemical. The most common of these devices is the pregnancy test, which yields a positive result when urine contains human chorionic gonadotropin, a hormone produced by the placenta. False positives are exceedingly rare with pregnancy tests, and when lab professionals want a quick result they sometimes use the disposable kits, which cost $8 to $18, instead of their huge $100,000 computer-driven analyzers.

BIOMEDICAL ENGINEER

Biomedical engineers are highly trained scientists who combine engineering and life science principles for research conducted on the biological aspects of animal and human life. They develop new theories, and modify and test existing theories on life systems. They design healthcare instruments and devices, or apply engineering principles to the study of human systems.

PREREQUISITES

Biomedical engineers should be highly motivated problem solvers. With so many interdisciplinary demands they need a broad educational background and familiarity with chemical, material, and electrical or mechanical engineering, as well as physiology and computers.

PREPARATION

Biomedical engineers need, minimally, an undergraduate degree in biomedical engineering or a related engineering field, and an advanced degree (preferably a Ph.D.) in some aspect of biomedical engineering.

PRINCIPAL DUTIES

Biomedical engineers are challenged to design medical instruments such as artificial organs, ultrasonic imagery devices, and systems to update hospital, laboratory, and clinical procedures. They also assist healthcare personnel in observing and treating physical disabilities and ailments.

ANOTHER WAY TO GET THERE

As a child, David Greene's favorite pastime was woodworking. In the years since then, Dr. Greene has found a way to use his manual dexterity to help others, and profoundly affect their lives, as well. Here's how:

The common thread throughout my life's choices has been my love of working with my hands. I always enjoyed building things and collecting tools, even if it interfered with what I was supposed to be doing—like schoolwork! I've also had a lifetime interest in the biological and life sciences, and for a while I wanted to be a veterinarian.

So when I graduated from high school in 1970, I enrolled at the University of Pennsylvania in a premed/prevet curriculum with a biology major. Of course I didn't give up the woodworking—I even found time to take a metalworking course. Eventually, though, I became disenchanted and dropped out.

I apprenticed with a cabinetmaker for a year or so, and then decided to start out on my own. My perfectionist nature got the better of me before long, though. I would estimate a job, then keep reworking it until I liked it, by which time I had dissipated any profit there might have been.

Through a series of coincidences—along with some family pressure—I returned to Penn, this time intending to become a dentist. One day, while in the gym working out, I overheard a conversation regarding research two people were doing—implanting materials in rabbits to test their biocompatibility for later use in humans.

I struck up a conversation with them, which eventually led to a research project from the Department of Orthopedics at the university hospital. Through it I built six instruments for use in hip replacement operations, two of which were totally new. This led me to a biomedical engineering major, and a job when I graduated—with the orthopedic division of Pfizer pharmaceuticals. One of my prosthetic innovations—which resulted in less distortion and a tighter fit—is being used in every knee prosthesis sold today.

Still, because my advancement at Pfizer depended on keeping up with meetings and management, I decided to leave. My family dentist finally convinced me that through dentistry I could merge my artistic and creative abilities, as well as help people. I applied to Harvard Dental School while I was still a biomedical engineer, and was accepted in the spring of 1978.

Today I specialize in the correction of jaw and facial deformities, the treatment of growth abnormalities, and the dental implants for the attachment or replacement of teeth, bridges, or dentures. I've changed a lot of people's lives for the better, which is a very gratifying feeling.

I also have some time for a little woodworking on the side—which is also a good feeling.

OUTLOOK

Between four and five thousand biomedical engineers are employed in hospitals, colleges and universities, medical and engineering schools, federal and state agencies, and private industry. It is expected that many more skilled biomedical engineers will be needed over the next several years to design computer applications and instrumentation, in addition to prosthetics and artificial organs.

EARNINGS

There is a wide range of earnings for biomedical engineers, depending on education and experience. Engineers in the federal government average about $40,000 a year; the average for college instructors is about $30,000, and full professors about $63,000. Those going into maxillofacial surgery and skilled designers in private industry can earn well into six figures.

Resource: **Biomedical Engineering Society**
P.O. Box 2399
Culver City, CA 90231

CHAPTER 11
Pursuing Careers in Mental Health

No other area of healthcare carries the mystery and misunderstanding that mental health does. Early Egyptian, Indian, Greek, and Roman writings show that the physicians who dealt with problems of human behavior regarded mental illnesses as a reflection of the gods' displeasure, or as evidence of demoniac possession. Most people today—physicians among them, fortunately—are considerably more enlightened.

Each year, nearly 41 million people suffer a diagnosable mental disorder ranging from mild depression to crippling schizophrenia. An additional 11 million will experience a substance use disorder. Meanwhile, work in the nation's laboratories continues to illuminate the causes and nature of mental illnesses, including the relationship of some disorders to chemical functions in the brain and to other medical illnesses. With this new knowledge, scientists are developing new diagnostic methods and treatments.

Disorders That Target Young Women

Each year millions of people in the United States are affected by three serious and sometimes life-threatening eating disorders—more than 90 percent of them adolescent and young adult women. One reason young women are vulnerable to eating disorders is that they tend to go on strict diets to achieve an "ideal" slender figure. Researchers say stringent dieting can play a key role in triggering eating disorders.

Anorexia nervosa involves extreme weight loss—at least 15 percent below a person's normal body weight. Anorexia victims look emaciated but are convinced they are overweight. Sometimes they must be hospitalized to prevent starvation. For reasons not yet fully understood, they become terrified of gaining weight.

Bulimia nervosa victims consume large amounts of food and then get rid of it by such means as vomiting, using laxatives, taking enemas, and exercising obsessively. Because many people with bulimia "binge and purge" in secret and maintain normal or above normal body weight, they often successfully hide their problem from others for years. Dental decay and esophygeal hernias are medical complications that can result from frequent vomiting.

Binge eating disorder is an illness that resembles bulimia nervosa because it is characterized by episodes of uncontrolled eating or binging. It differs from bulimia because its sufferers do not purge their bodies of excess food. People with binge eating disorder feel that they lose control of themselves when eating. They eat large quantities of food and do not stop until they are uncomfortably full. Most people with the disorder are obese and have a history of weight fluctuation.

Treatment can save the life of someone with an eating disorder. Friends, relatives, teachers, and physicians all play an important role in helping the ill person start—and stay with—a treatment program. Call local hospitals or university medical centers to find out about eating disorder clinics, or write: Information Resources and Inquiries Branch, National Institute of Mental Health, 5600 Fishers Lane, Room 7C-02, Rockville, MD 20857.

PSYCHIATRIST

Psychiatrists diagnose and treat patients with mental, emotional, and behavioral disorders. They are trained to understand the body's functions and the complex relationship between emotional illness and other medical illnesses. A psychiatrist is the mental health professional and physician best qualified to distinguish between physical and psychological causes of both mental and physical distress. Psychiatrists organize data on a patient's family, medical history, and the onset of symptoms obtained from the patient, relatives, nurses, and social workers. Psychiatrists examine patients to determine their general physical condition. They order laboratory and other special diagnostic tests, and evaluate the data obtained. They determine the nature of the mental disorder, formulate a treatment program, and use a variety of psychotherapeutic methods and medications to treat the patient.

PREREQUISITES

Students need outstanding intelligence to complete the required studies, as well as perseverance and good health to survive the long training period. Psychiatrists must be emotionally stable to deal with patients objectively, and they must be good listeners.

PREPARATION

Like other physicians-in-training (see Chapter 2, Career Opportunities as Doctors), students of psychiatry work in several specialty rotations after attaining their M.D. or D.O. In the first year they may work in internal medicine or pediatrics. Then they work for three years in a psychiatric hospital or a general hospital's psychiatric ward. Psychiatrists who wish to become psychoanalysts spend six years in part-time training, either during or after residency, and also undergo psychoanalysis themselves during this period.

PRINCIPAL DUTIES

The treatment a psychiatrist employs depends on the patient's needs. In some cases the psychiatrist may refer the patient to another psychiatrist who specializes in a recommended treatment or sub-specialty.

Some psychiatrists have general practices, treating patients with a variety of mental disorders. Others specialize in certain types of clients. Three sub-specialties recognized by the American Medical Association are *addiction psychiatry* (focusing on the prevention, evaluation, and treatment of substance abuse and dependence); *child and adolescent psychiatry;* and *geriatric psychiatry.*

OUTLOOK

Opportunities for both private practice and salaried psychiatrists is expected to be excellent through the rest of this decade. There is a particular shortage of psychiatrists in rural areas and public institutions.

EARNINGS

The median net income of psychiatrists, after expenses, is about $120,000 annually—allowing for differences by region and setting. Those in private practice, for example, average somewhat more; and those in salaried, public institutions (such as clinics and state hospitals) can average considerably less.

    Resource: Office of Education
                       American Psychiatric Association
                       1400 K Street, NW
                       Washington, DC 20037
                       (career and education information)

PSYCHIATRIC TECHNICIAN

Psychiatric technicians and other mental health workers provide nursing care and participate in treatment programs for mentally ill, emotionally disturbed, or mentally retarded patients in psychiatric hospitals or mental health clinics. The job description for psychiatric technician may be applicable in varying degrees to similar mental health support positions with other titles, depending on the nomenclature in your state or region. If you are interested in a mental health support position, investigate also such titles as "mental health associate," "mental health assistant," or "case manager."

PREREQUISITES

Psychiatric technicians need stable personalities, the ability to relate well to people, and the motivation to help others. Patience and understanding are required in working with people who may be disagreeable because of their illness. The ability to remain calm in emergencies and a strong sense of responsibility are two other essential characteristics.

PREPARATION

Psychiatric technicians must have two years of training beyond high school. Interested students should find out as early as possible in high school about the requirements of schools they want to attend, to assure meeting all courses mandated. The two-year post-high school training program usually leads to an associate of arts or associate of science degree. High school students should take biology and, if available, psychology and sociology. Program courses include anatomy, physiology, basic nursing, and medical science. Most health technology programs emphasize interviewing skills so that, on the job, technicians will be able to correctly read tones of voice and shades of meaning regarding what people say and do, and be able to observe and record the behavior people exhibit. Graduates from mental health technology programs usually can choose from a variety of job possibilities.

PRINCIPAL DUTIES

Psychiatric technicians work under the supervision of psychiatrists, psychologists, registered nurses, or more senior psychiatric technicians. Their duties consist of both nursing responsibilities and assisting in treatment programs. Nursing duties can include helping patients with bathing and keeping their beds, clothing, and living areas clean; administering oral medications and hypodermic injections according to physician prescriptions; and recording readings of patients' pulse, temperature, and respiration rates. Their treatment program assistance can include leading individual and group therapy sessions, and observing behavior patterns of patients and reporting their observations to medical and psychiatric staff members.

OUTLOOK

A trend toward shorter periods of hospitalization is expected to lead to the development of more comprehensive community health centers, increasing the need for psychiatric technicians in outpatient settings. Also, concerns about rising healthcare costs should lead to psychiatric technicians taking over more functions traditionally held by higher-paid professionals.

EARNINGS

Entry-level salaries for workers holding an associate's degree usually range from about $11,500 to about $21,000. Many senior psychiatric technicians earn more than $33,000 yearly.

        Resource: **American Psychiatric Association**
                                  1400 K Street NW
                                  Washington, DC 20005

"Decade of the Brain"

The President and Congress have declared the 1990s "The Decade of the Brain," to draw attention to mental disorders such as depression, manic-depressive illness, schizophrenia, panic disorder, and obsessive-compulsive disorder. Through continuing research in animals and humans, doctors and scientists hope to use the knowledge gained to develop new therapies and help more people overcome mental illness.

PSYCHOLOGIST

Psychology is the scientific discipline that studies mental processes and behavior in humans and other animals. Psychologists study human behavior to understand, explain, and change people's behavior. They may apply psychological treatments to a variety of medical and surgical conditions or provide mental health services in hospitals, clinics, or private settings. Psychologists also work in a large number of nonhealthcare areas.

PREREQUISITES

More so than in most professions, aspiring psychologists interested in direct patient care must be emotionally stable, mature, sensitive, compassionate, and be able to deal effectively with people. Patience and perseverance are also desirable characteristics, because results from treatment often can be a long time in coming.

PREPARATION

A doctoral degree is generally required for employment as a psychologist. Those with a Ph.D. qualify for a wide range of teaching, research, clinical, and counseling positions.

People with a master's degree in psychology can administer tests as psychological assistants. Under supervision of doctoral level psychologists, they can conduct research in laboratories, complete evaluations, counsel patients, or perform administrative duties. They may teach in high schools or two-year colleges, or work as school psychologists or counselors.

A bachelor's degree in psychology qualifies a person to assist psychologists and other professionals in community mental health centers and vocational rehabilitation offices. Without additional academic training, however, advancement possibilities are severely limited.

PRINCIPAL DUTIES

Clinical psychologists, who constitute the largest specialty, generally work in independent or group practice or in hospitals or clinics. They help mentally or emotionally disturbed people adjust to life, and are increasingly helping all kinds of medical and surgical patients deal with their illnesses or injuries. They may also work in physical medicine and rehabilitation settings, treating patients with spinal cord injuries, chronic pain or illness, stroke, arthritis, or neurologic conditions such as multiple sclerosis.

Health psychologists promote good health through health maintenance counseling programs designed to help people stop smoking or lose weight.

Death Education

I was living in a distant town when my father died alone. Four years later I was still racked with guilt and anger—guilt for not having been there, anger for the distressing way he died. I knew I had to work out these issues in a proactive way.

It was at this time I discovered the Hospice Movement, and through a local agency realized this was a philosophy I wanted to explore. The eight-week training program was not only a thorough exploration of death and dying, but an effective life skills evaluation course. When I completed it, I decided to volunteer as a bereavement counselor.

After additional training, seminars and conferences—and the support of a wonderful program director—I began to lead my own groups, specializing in therapy for teenagers. Teens need to talk about what's happening in their lives, but death is usually too scary for their friends to deal with, and more often than not family members are too absorbed in their own pain to help. It's very satisfying to help these young people learn to cope with and move through the tragedy they are facing.

Death educators are often hired to present education programs in various settings: schools, hospitals, and community organizations, for example. As the topic of death and dying becomes more open in our culture, there will be a greater need for education about it.

For more information, contact: Dorothy Meinhold, Natural Death Education Center, Mt. Ida College, Newton, Massachusetts 02205.

OUTLOOK

Employment of psychologists is expected to grow much faster than the average for all occupations through the year 2005. An increased emphasis on mental health maintenance in conjunction with the treatment of physical illness will contribute in part to this increased employment.

EARNINGS

Annual median salary for psychologists with doctoral degrees is approximately $48,000 in counseling psychology and $53,000 in clinical psychology. The median annual salary of master's degree holders was $37,000 in counseling psychology and $40,000 in clinical psychology. Some psychologists have much higher earnings, especially those in private practice.

    Resource: **American Psychological Association**
                      Education in Psychology and Accreditation Offices
                      750 First Street NE
                      Washington, DC 20002

MENTAL HEALTH SOCIAL WORKER

PREREQUISITES

Social workers should be emotionally mature, objective, and sensitive to people and their problems. They must be able to handle responsibility, work independently, and maintain good working relationships with clients and coworkers.

PREPARATION

A bachelor's degree is the minimum requirement for most positions. Besides the bachelor's in social work (BSW), undergraduate majors in psychology, sociology, and related fields satisfy hiring requirements in some agencies, especially those in small communities. A master's degree in social work (MSW) is generally necessary for positions in health and mental health settings. Some social workers go into private practice. Most private practitioners are clinical social workers who provide psychotherapeutic counseling, usually paid through health insurance. Private practitioners must have completed an MSW and a period of supervised work experience.

PRINCIPAL DUTIES

Mental health social workers provide services for persons with mental or emotional problems, such as individual or group therapy, outreach, crisis intervention, social rehabilitation, and training in skills of everyday living. They may also help plan for supportive services to ease patients' return to the community.

ANOTHER WAY TO GET THERE

Kathleen Rooney's decision to go into medical social work wasn't the realization of a childhood dream, but rather a way to deal with her life at a crucial crossroad. Here's how she describes it:

In my mid-forties, a personal crisis forced me to reevaluate my life and career options. I'd been a teacher, a wife, and a mother of three children. After several attempts at a new career, and with the encouragement of several friends who were social workers, I came to the conclusion that my life experiences, my interpersonal skills, and my interest in social issues would be a good fit with social work.

In 1982 I entered graduate school. Many of my classmates were already "in the field" working on a master's degree. This was somewhat intimidating at first, but clearly I had much to offer and draw upon, and the learning experience was challenging and energizing. When I received my master's (30 years after receiving my bachelor's!), the sense of accomplishment was exquisite.

Although my knowledge of hospitals had been limited to my childbirth experiences, that is the setting for my years as a social worker. A hospital is a fast-paced, complex, rapidly changing work environment. Each day brings new, unknown experiences. I see myself as a generalist, using my clinical skills to work with people who are in crisis due to hospitalization. I am part of the healthcare team working toward the best possible outcome for patients and their families.

People do not come to me. I go to them—whether in a hospital room, a lobby, an emergency room, or a family waiting room. I assess, provide information, counsel, listen, facilitate, intervene—always trying to respect the needs of those with whom I am working. One needs to be self-directed, flexible, creative, have a sense of humor about oneself, and be aware of one's limitations.

This profession has taught me so much about what it is to be strong and courageous. I've shared people's joy and sadness in their times of triumph and defeat. Of the many doors that have been opened to me in my life, I'm glad I walked through the one marked "Social Work."

OUTLOOK

Employment of social workers is expected to increase faster than the average for all occupations through the year 2005. Requirements for social workers will grow with increases in the need for and concern about services to the mentally ill, the mentally retarded, and individuals and families in crisis.

EARNINGS

The median earnings of social workers with MSW degrees is a little over $30,000. For those with BSW degrees, earnings average just over $20,000.

Resources: **National Association of Social Workers**
750 First Street NE, Suite 700
Washington, DC 20002
(career information)

Council on Social Work Education
1600 Duke Street, Suite 300
Alexandria, VA 22314

CERTIFIED ALCOHOL AND DRUG ABUSE COUNSELOR

Certified alcohol and drug abuse counselors (CADACs) work with clients individually and in group settings regarding addiction and relapse prevention. They assess and evaluate clients for the purpose of making recommendations for further drug or alcohol abuse treatment. They maintain case records and prepare reports of work accomplished and work planned. CADAC workers attend meetings and collaborate with treatment facility personnel. They document data and activities, and undergo additional training as required.

To become a certified alcohol and drug abuse counselor in most states, applicants must have approximately three years' experience—often expressed as "hours of supervised counseling." For example, the state of New Hampshire requires a total of 6,000 hours for certification: 2,000 hours in the alcohol area, 2,000 hours in drugs other than alcohol, and 2,000 in the "alcohol and other drug abuse" area. All experience must have been obtained within the eight years immediately before applying for certification.

The National Certification Examination is conducted quarterly in March, June, September, and December. A registration form and candidate guide are available at no charge. Applicants may also request a study guide at a cost of $24.95.

The annual salary for an experienced CADAC is from $21,000 to $35,000.

Resource:	National Organization for Human Service Education
Brookdale Community College
Lyncroft, NJ 07730
(certification application information)

OUTREACH WORKER

Outreach workers need a high school diploma or GED (although most have undergraduate degrees). They must be 21 years of age or older, and have extensive knowledge of substance abuse, drugs of choice, methods of administering, and treatment facilities and be indigenous to and respected by the population being served. Those workers recovering from dependency must be stable in recovery for at least three years or more. Outreach workers are supervised by a program coordinator. Basic objectives are to provide information and skills to effect behavioral changes, both to draw the medically underserved into the system and to decrease substance abusers' risk of acquiring or transmitting HIV and related diseases.

The annual salary for an experienced outreach worker ranges from $14,000 to approximately $25,000.

Resource:	National Health Careers Information Hotline
Thomas Jefferson University College of Allied Sciences
Philadelphia, PA 19107

PROFESSIONAL COUNSELOR

Professional counselors help people meet personal, social, educational, and career-related challenges. They provide individual counseling, group counseling, testing and evaluation, for example, or a combination of these services. Areas of expertise include career counseling, measurement and testing, marriage and families, substance abuse, rehabilitation, mental health counseling, and student and adult development. Professional counselors are employed in hospitals, mental health facilities, rehabilitation centers, schools and universities, correctional facilities, and private and nonprofit organizations.

PREREQUISITES

Students need good verbal skills and at least an average ability in mathematics. Although professional counselors are required to work with facts and collect information about clients, anyone interested in counseling should be able to work well with people, either independently or as part of a group.

PREPARATION

Professional counselors are expected to have obtained a master's degree from an accredited program and extensive approved supervisory training with direct client contact. A significant number of professional counselors have a specialized degree or a doctorate. General training requirements may differ depending on the type of counseling practiced and the employment location. In 42 states and the District of Columbia, professional counselors must be licensed to practice. Many counselors also choose to become nationally certified by the National Board for Certified Counselors, which offers a National Certified Counselor credential and specialty certification in career, gerontology, school, clinical mental health, and addiction counseling. Counselors must take continuing education classes and workshops to maintain their license and certification.

PRINCIPAL DUTIES

Professional counselors devote time to collecting, organizing, and synthesizing information about clients, using records, a variety of assessment instruments, and interviews. This process of information gathering is followed by helping clients to cope with physical or emotional concerns; to combat substance abuse and eating disorders; to resolve personal and family conflicts, such as death, abuse, or sexuality concerns; and to develop preventive life skills for dealing with transition and change. Many professional counselors focus on prevention and development, intervening before a concern or problem becomes a crisis.

OUTLOOK

Employment of professional counselors is expected to grow significantly through the year 2005. Opportunities overall should be excellent, with available positions expected to grow by 26 percent. In some areas of the United States the increase in available jobs is expected to reach 37 to 40 percent.

EARNINGS

Nationally, the average salary for experienced professional counselors is approximately $3,350 per month. Salaries for entry-level counselors average just over $2,000 per month. Self-employed counselors and those working for private companies—or who have well-established private practices—often earn more than the average.

Resource: **American Counseling Association**
5999 Stevenson Avenue
Alexandria, VA 22304

CHAPTER 12
Pursuing Careers in Speech-Language Pathology

Most people take hearing, speech, and language for granted. We speak to family, friends, colleagues, and strangers. Those who don't take these facilities for granted either have a communication disorder themselves or are close to someone else who does.

Forty-two million Americans—one person out of every six—have a communication disorder. Two thirds of these are hearing impaired. (One baby out of every 1,000 is born deaf.) The other 14 million have a voice, speech, or language disorder. Each can be helped in some way by a speech-language pathologist or audiologist; or by a speech, language, or hearing scientist. All of these professionals evaluate, treat, and conduct research into human communication and its disorders.

SPEECH-LANGUAGE PATHOLOGIST

Speech-language pathologists (SLPs) identify, assess, and treat various disorders caused by conditions such as hearing loss, emotional problems, mental retardation, cerebral palsy, and brain damage. Speech-language pathologists are sometimes called speech clinicians or speech therapists.

PREREQUISITES

Working as a speech-language pathologist requires attention to detail and intense concentration. The emotional needs of clients and their families may be demanding. Slow or no client progress can be extremely frustrating. And even the slightest progress must be observed and recorded so that applicable treatment adjustments, however minor, can be implemented.

PREPARATION

A master's degree in speech-language pathology is the standard credential. All 43 states that regulate this field require a master's degree or equivalent. In some states, speech-language bachelor's degree holders are allowed to work in schools. These people usually must be certified by the state educational agency, and are classified as special education teachers rather than speech-language pathologists. About 230 colleges and universities offer master's programs in speech-language pathology.

ANOTHER WAY TO GET THERE

Janet Davis, M.S., C.C.C., S.L.P., knew early in life that she wanted to go into the healthcare field. Here she traces her career plans as a youngster, and how she translated them into reality:

My interest in the field of speech-language pathology was influenced strongly by my parents. My mother is an English and foreign language teacher, and my father is an obstetrician-gynecologist. I knew early in high school that I wanted a career in a "helping" profession. Yet I did not want to be a teacher or a nurse.

In college I volunteered at a rehabilitation institute specializing in the evaluation and treatment of traumatically brain-injured children. That introduced me to neurology, brain function, and brain recovery following trauma—and by my junior year I had decided that a speech-language pathologist was the perfect combination of a teacher and a doctor. But there were a few interim goals I had to attain first, such as:
- Bachelor's degree in speech-language pathology
- Master's degree in speech-language pathology
- Nine-month Clinical Fellowship Year
- Pass national examination
- Certificate of Clinical Competence
- State SLP license (in nearly all states)

Working in a K–12 public school system, my "typical day" begins at 8:00 a.m. and ends at 3:00 or 3:30 p.m. I usually see students for treatment in 30-minute sessions, in or outside the classroom setting. I meet with them individually or in groups of two or three. All treatment settings are determined after careful evaluation of the pupil's needs.

The speech-language pathologist is responsible for:
- Initial and discharge evaluations
- Three-year re-evaluations (mandated by the state)
- Monthly progress reports
- Writing a treatment plan or intervention as part of the student's individualized education plan

- Treating the students
- Meeting with parents, educators, and other health professionals
- Revising treatment plans on an ongoing basis

Additional responsibilities include community inservices and maintaining continuing education units by attending workshops and professional seminars, both in-state and nationwide.

Referrals for evaluation may be generated by parents, physicians, teachers, and other allied health professionals (for example, nurses, physical therapists, and occupational therapists).

Evaluations consist of both standardized and informal test measurements. Evaluations require from two to six hours, depending on the age and attention span of the student, the nature of the disability, the number of test batteries given, scoring time, and report writing. Based on the evaluation results, we are able to set our therapy goals and put together a treatment plan. Oh yes, we also need to build in time for note writing, responding to parent phone calls, and meeting with other team members, to round out our "typical" day.

Under this "inclusionary model," the student benefits from a virtually seamless continuum of services. The SLP works in the classroom with the student, usually plus a teacher's aide; the aide accompanies the student to a one-on-one therapy session and comes back to the classroom with new ideas for improving communication. The SLP is thus able to train other staff members to carry out therapy goals throughout the student's day.

Student progress is sometimes visible only after months of work. To watch a multiple-handicapped student bring a spoon to his mouth to feed himself, or smile and vocalize in response to a familiar voice or sound is an enormously gratifying experience, especially after weeks or months of trying to achieve such a seemingly simple goal. Another great reward of working as an SLP in a school setting is the teamwork and support of the other teachers and professionals.

I think two of the attributes most important to being an effective SLP are open-mindedness and flexibility. Strong verbal, writing, and organizational skills—and, of course, patience—also promote efficiency.

Some years ago I went through a frightening experience while under anesthesia. I knew what was going on around me because I could hear, but I was unable to communicate what I was feeling to the doctors and nurses who were right there! At that moment I was able to identify with the way I know some of my students feel. I have worked with so many people who have the desire and intelligence to communicate but who have been robbed of the means to do so.

It is important to realize that speech-language pathologists don't cure—they facilitate. We facilitate one of life's most vital, yet taken for granted processes: communication.

PRINCIPAL DUTIES

Speech-language pathologists work in a number of settings, among them: public and private schools, hospitals and rehabilitation centers, nursing care facilities, colleges and universities, private practice offices, state and local health departments, home health agencies, long-term facilities, adult day-care centers, research laboratories, and private industry. Speech clinicians provide services to infants and children, adolescents and adults, and older people.

Speech clinicians render assistance:
- To those who stutter, to increase fluency
- To victims of stroke or brain tumor, to regain language, speech, or swallowing ability
- To families of patients, to help them cope with a family member's disorder
- To individuals and community, to advise on ways to prevent speech and language disorders
- With developing proper control of the vocal and respiratory systems for correct voice production
- To teach individuals to use alternative means of communication

Although speech and language professionals work closely with teachers, physicians, psychologists, social workers, rehabilitation counselors, and other members of an interdisciplinary team, they are autonomous and do not work under direct medical supervision.

OUTLOOK

Employment for speech-language pathologists is expected to grow much faster than the average for all occupations. In 1995, *Money* magazine listed it eleventh in a survey of the "Fifty Hottest Jobs." An aging population is one contributory factor, increasing the number of those affected by hearing loss, strokes, and other communication disorders.

EARNINGS

Median annual salary for a full-time salaried speech-language pathologist is just under $40,000. Those with Ph.D.s reported a median annual salary of nearly $50,000. (Median annual salaries were computed from combined academic- and 1995 calendar-year based salaries.)

Resource:	**American Speech-Language-Hearing Association**
	Membership, Career Development Division
	10801 Rockville Pike
	Rockville, MD 20852

Language and Languages

Ursula Bellugi is a pioneer in studying sign language to identify those parts of the brain that handle linguistic tasks. Her research, collected from various languages, suggests that human language capacity may be genetically determined.

AUDIOLOGIST

Prerequisites, educational requirements, employment outlook and prospective earnings are almost identical to those of speech-language pathologists. The job description can vary, however, in those infrequent situations where the two functions do not overlap.

PRINCIPAL DUTIES

Audiologists work with people who have hearing and related problems. They use audiometers and other testing devices to measure the decibal level at which a person begins to hear sounds and the ability to distinguish among sounds, and they perform tests to determine the nature and extent of hearing loss. Audiologists may coordinate these results with medical, educational, and psychological information, make a diagnosis, and determine a course of treatment. The treatment may include examining and cleaning the ear canal, fitting a hearing aid, auditory training, and instruction in speech or lip-reading. Audiologists may recommend the use of amplifiers and alerting devices. They also test noise levels in workplaces and conduct hearing protection programs.

Audiologists may also:
- Serve as consultants to government and industry on environmental and noise-induced hearing loss
- Initiate hearing conservation programs in industry and with the public to prevent hearing loss from occupational or environmental noise exposure

OUTLOOK

Identical to that for speech-language pathologist: extremely favorable for the next several years.

EARNINGS

The median salary for audiologists on a calendar-year basis is a little over $40,000. Those audiologists with doctoral degrees can expect a median annual salary of about $60,000.

Resource: American Speech-Language-Hearing Association
10801 Rockville Pike
Rockville, MD 10852

CHAPTER 13

Pursuing Careers in Pharmacy

Pharmacy is concerned with the preparation, distribution, and use of drugs prescribed by doctors, dentists, and other practitioners. As a profession, pharmacy grew slowly in the United States until 1906, when the Federal Pure Food and Drug Act was passed. For the past 65 years or so, all pharmaceuticals and drugs sold in the United States have had to be approved by the Food and Drug Administration (FDA). The work of the pharmacist has become increasingly important since then, largely because of the potential danger from side effects of the thousands of drugs now on the market. Actually, the "compounding" function—mixing the ingredients to form powders, tablets, capsules, ointments, and solutions—is less a part of a pharmacist's job these days, because most medicines are produced by pharmaceutical companies in standard dosage and form.

PHARMACIST

PREREQUISITES

Pharmacists require a combination of skills and attributes, depending on the setting in which they work. They need to be able to compound and dispense a wide variety of prescriptions accurately. For this they need both scientific aptitude and manual dexterity. Those pharmacists dealing with the public need good interpersonal skills, as well. Those owning their own businesses should have a good entrepreneurial sense.

PREPARATION

A license to practice pharmacy is required in all 50 states. To get the license, one needs a degree from an accredited college of pharmacy, and then must pass a state exam and serve an internship under a licensed pharmacist. Many pharmacists are licensed to practice in more than one state, and most states require continuing education to justify license renewal.

Seventy-five U.S. colleges and schools of pharmacy offer accredited professional degree programs, most requiring one or two years of college-level pre-pharmacy education. Sixty-three schools offer graduate programs in the pharmaceutical sciences at the master's or doctoral level.

At least five years of study after high school are required for an accredited bachelor of science degree. A doctor of pharmacy (Pharm.D.) normally requires six years, during which an intervening bachelor's degree is not awarded. Entry requirements usually include mathematics, chemistry, biology, and physics, as well as courses in the social sciences. Although a bachelor's degree is sufficient for most community practices, a growing number of hospitals prefer a Pharm.D. degree.

For pharmacy students in financial need, a wide range of grants, scholarships, and loans are available. For further information, contact the Interorganizational Council on Student Affairs, 2215 Constitution Avenue, NW, Washington, DC 20037. (See also the Bibliography section: Scholarships, Grants, and Low-Cost Loans.)

Ethnopharmacy
(From a review by Byron Bailey of Mark Plotkin's *Tales of a Shaman's Apprentice* in the January 25, 1995 issue of the *Journal of the AMA*)

Throughout history, the shaman has been a figure of power and mystery. In South America, the shaman was second only to the chief in tribunal authority and importance. Even today, he serves as physician, priest, pharmacist, and psychiatrist.

The shaman contacts the spirit world to diagnose an illness and to determine the most effective treatment. This usually involves the selection of a plant, then boiling portions of it to make a therapeutic tea. Similar remedies have proven effective for comparable illnesses across widely separated cultures. For example, quinine is derived from the bark of the cinchona tree and was discovered thousands of years ago by separate Indian tribes in what is now Ecuador and Peru.

* * *

(From an article by Robert A. Hamilton in *Connecticut* magazine, March 1996)

A steady stream of strange packages from around the world has been arriving at pharmaceutical giant Pfizer lately, and the company—with over $10 billion thanks to drugs such as Procardia, Zoloft, and Enablex—makes no secret of its renewed emphasis on plants as potential sources for new medicines. It has dispatched emissaries to sites as diverse as South American rain forests and Connecticut highway medians to search for shrubs, flowers, bark, and roots that might hold a cure for cancer, depression, or diabetes. In the last two years the company has tested more than 1,000 species of plants.

PRINCIPAL DUTIES

Pharmacists in retail pharmacies answer customer questions about both prescription and over-the-counter drugs—their possible adverse reactions, for example—and make recommendations after asking their own questions about customer susceptibility to certain drugs, and current medication schedules.

Pharmacists in hospitals and clinics advise the medical staff on the selection and effects of drugs, in addition to dispensing medications. Pharmacists who work in home healthcare prepare medications for use in the home and monitor drug therapy.

Most pharmacists keep computerized records of patients' drug therapies to assure that harmful drug interactions are avoided. Some pharmacists specialize in specific aspects of drug therapy, such as drugs for psychiatric disorders or intravenous nutrition.

OUTLOOK

About three out of five of the 168,000 pharmacists today work in community pharmacies, either independently owned, part of a drugstore chain, or part of a grocery or department store. Employment is expected to grow faster than the average for all occupations for the next several years. Scientific advances will likely make more drug products available, for one thing. Also, new developments in administering medication will broaden the usage base.

EARNINGS

Median annual earnings of full-time, salaried pharmacists are a little over $53,000. The bottom 10 percent earned $31,500, and the top 10 percent about $75,000. Pharmacists employed by chain drug stores, supermarkets, discount stores, and HMOs receive more benefits than those in independent drug stores. Pharmacist-owners tend to earn considerably more than salaried pharmacists.

> Resource: American Association of Colleges of Pharmacy
> 1426 Prince Street
> Alexandria, VA 22314
> (Career and educational information)

ANOTHER WAY TO GET THERE

George Bowersox decided on a career in pharmacy when he was a high school student working as a retail clerk. Here he answers questions about himself and his work, describing a typical day in the life of a pharmacist and what attracted him to the profession:

What are your primary duties as a pharmacist?

As a community retail pharmacist, my prime reponsibility is to take prescriptions from the physician, either in writing or by phone. After receiving the prescription, I have the following additional responsibilities:
- To check the patient's medication history and do a drug review
- To check that the dosage is appropriate for the condition
- To look for any contraindications (allergies) and drug overlap
- To check for any drug interactions with other medications
- To check that the prescription meets all federal and state requirements for dispensing

- To check that the prescription meets the patient's insurance requirements

After performing these checks, I prepare a label so the medication can be dispensed to the patient. The label includes directions for proper use and storage of the prescription, as well as any applicable advisory labels. I offer to counsel the patient and answer any questions regarding the prescription. I make myself available to recommend over-the-counter medications to treat all kinds of ailments. I also refer the patient to appropriate doctors, dentists, and other healthcare providers, as may be indicated.

What drew you to your profession?
I decided to be a pharmacist after working in a community pharmacy as a retail clerk. The biggest reason is that I saw how much respect and trust the pharmacist had in the community. I also liked the flexible hours: The days are long, but there are more days off than average. The salary is very respectable for someone just out of school. It just doesn't progress a lot from there.

What are the greatest challenges and rewards of your job?
The greatest challenge is very basic. As a pharmacist you must be infallible. There is no margin for error. Any mistake could result in extreme consequences to a patient's health.

The part of the job I find most rewarding is the role of educator. I enjoy informing the patient about the use of medication, and diagnosing many of their initial problems. I see many people before they go to their physician, and they trust my judgment regarding their health. I also enjoy being part of a profession that gets the highest ratings for trust and honesty in Gallup polls year after year.

PHARMACIST ASSISTANT

A pharmacist assistant mixes and dispenses prescribed medicines and pharmaceutical preparations in the absence of or under the supervision of a registered pharmacist. Other duties include issuing medicine, labeling and storing supplies, and cleaning equipment and work areas. (If this career path interests you, ask your local pharmacist to spend a few minutes describing the duties to you. It may lead to an after-school job that puts you on the right track!) About 52,000 pharmacy assistants are employed nationwide, with the growth projection over the next several years faster than average.

The Childproof Safety Cap: A Response to Need

In the 1940s, when flavored "baby aspirin" first came on the market, children ate the pills like candy and aspirin overdoses soared. Dr. Jay Arena, a North Carolina pediatrician and expert in poison control, called an aspirin manufacturer to see what could be done. Their work together led to production of the first childproof safety caps.

Dr. Arena also suggested reducing the dosage for children's aspirin and the amount of aspirin in each package. His ideas are credited with helping to cut the fatal aspirin overdose rate among children from 25 percent of all poisoning deaths then to the 1 percent it is today.

CHAPTER 14

Pursuing Careers in Physical or Occupational Therapy

Those of you looking for a healthcare career solely on the number of job openings available need read no further. In Chapter 1, you learned that 11 of the top 30 fastest-growing jobs in the United States were to be found in the healthcare industry. As it happens, four of these 11 jobs are in the field of physical and occupational therapy. Here is the good news, based on percentage of job growth expected to occur between 1992 and 2005, according to a Bureau of Labor Statistics study:
- Physical and corrective therapist assistants—93 percent
- Physical therapists—88 percent
- Occupational therapist assistants—78 percent
- Occupational therapists—60 percent

PHYSICAL THERAPIST

As has been true in other areas of medical treatment, combat medical teams in World War II and the Korean and Vietnamese wars contributed significantly to improving the rehabilitation of seriously injured soldiers, leading to the acceptance of many modern physical therapy practices. Today physical therapy has expanded beyond hospitals. Many physical therapists now work in private practices, nursing homes, home health agencies, sports facilities, and in private homes.

Physical therapists' patients consist of recovering accident victims, people disabled by neurological disorders such as multiple sclerosis and cerebral palsy, and post-operative patients of all ages recovering full or partial use of parts of their bodies. Therapists improve patients' mobility, relieve pain, and prevent or limit permanent physical disabilities to whatever extent possible.

PREREQUISITES

Physical therapists should be patient, persuasive, emotionally stable, and tactful in helping patients to understand their treatment and adjust to their disabilities. Similar traits are needed to deal effectively with patients' families. They should also have manual dexterity and physical stamina. On any given day they will stoop, kneel, crouch, lift, and stand for long periods of time. They must frequently lift their patients, or help them stand or walk.

PREPARATION

All states require physical therapists to pass a licensing exam after completing an accredited physical therapy program. Entry level education in physical therapy is available in 65 bachelor's degree and 80 master's degree programs. The bachelor's degree program includes basic science courses such as biology, chemistry, and physics, and moves on to biomechanics, neuroanatomy, human growth and development, and therapeutic procedures. Besides classroom and lab instruction, students receive supervised clinical experience in hospitals. A master's degree is of value to students interested in administrative and teaching positions.

PRINCIPAL DUTIES

Physical therapists evaluate patients' medical history; test and measure their strength, range of motion, and ability to function; and develop written treatment plans, based primarily on physician instructions. As treatment continues, they document progress, conduct periodic re-evaluations, and modify treatment accordingly. Treatment usually includes exercise, stretching, and manipulating stiff joints and unused muscles. Later in the treatment, therapists encourage patients to exercise muscles on their own to further increase strength, flexibility, and range of motion.

Physical therapists also use electrical stimulation, heat, cold, or ultrasound to relieve pain, improve the condition of muscles or related tissues, or to reduce swelling. They may use traction or deep-tissue massage to relieve pain and restore function. Therapists also teach and motivate patients to use crutches, prostheses, and wheelchairs to perform day-to-day activities. They also demonstrate at-home exercises. Some therapists are generalists; others specialize in such areas as pediatrics, geriatrics, orthopedics, sports therapy, or sometimes specific parts of the body.

Animal Therapists

Chenny Troupe, Inc. is a Chicago-based volunteer organization that supplies dogs to people who use animals to help motivate them with required physical activity. Walking with them, throwing toys to them, or even giving verbal commands, for example, helps stroke-recovery patients.

* * *

Horseback riding is an exhilarating, freeing experience for children who are usually confined to wheelchairs or trapped by other disabilities. The North American Riding for the Handicapped Association has many accredited facilities that offer riding for disabled children.

OUTLOOK

Employment of physical therapists is expected to grow much faster than the average for all occupations through the year 2005. As new medical technologies save more people, these additional people will need therapy. A rapidly growing elderly population is exceptionally susceptible to chronic and debilitating conditions that can be relieved with therapy. There have been shortages of physical therapists in recent years, which further accentuates the current need for qualified people.

EARNINGS

The median annual salary of full-time physical therapists is about $37,600. The top 10 percent earn about $61,800, and the bottom 10 percent earn just under $20,000.

Resource:	American Physical Therapy Association
1111 N. Fairfax Street
Alexandria, VA 22314

ANOTHER WAY TO GET THERE

To paraphrase an old saying, "Some people are born into a career, some seek one out, and some have a career thrust upon them." As physical therapist Sean Gallagher sees it, his story falls into the last category.

A career in physical therapy was the furthest thing from my mind when I was a kid. I left home when I was seventeen and went out West to Montana, where I worked on a ranch for a while. Later I built houses, was a plumber, worked as an excavator—that kind of stuff.

Finally I decided I wanted to go to college with a theater major. I started out at the University of Montana, studying modern dance, and I loved it. My teacher said I needed more advanced instruction than U.M. could offer. He recommended that I transfer to his old college, Temple University, which happens to be in my hometown of Philadelphia.

Physical Therapist

At age twenty-one, I entered Temple as a dance major. It all went great—I was busy with my studies, and now and then I'd have a semi-pro dance gig for money. Then, bad luck; in my third year of school I suffered a lower back injury. The doctor recommended lots of rest, which really annoyed me. I didn't want just a band-aid treatment; I was looking for recovery. Asking around, I discovered that there were no physical therapists available who were skilled working with dancers. And that's when I added a second major to my studies: physical therapy.

As my back got better, I started dancing again. Unfortunately, the pain never went away, and the stress of dancing just made it worse. I realized that my dream of becoming a professional dancer was over—and that if I continued I could end up badly crippled. It was a heart-breaking decision. A big help to me, though, was the pleasure I was getting from the physical therapy training.

By wonderful good luck, my clinical instructor and mentor was Marika Molnar, now looked on as a pioneer in performing-arts physical therapy. Working with her, I treated dancers in the New York City Ballet company. After graduation in 1986, I began a full-time practice with the Pennsylvania Ballet.

From personal experience, as well as my work with two ballet companies, I knew just how valuable the services of a physical therapist could be. I finally decided to make this my life work. By 1988 I was in New York treating professional dancers full-time, and in 1990 I opened my office, Performing Arts Physical Therapy. Since then I've joined with former Temple classmates to add two more offices, in Seattle and Los Angeles.

My experience as a dancer has worked as a huge advantage for me. I've "walked the walk," you know, and that makes for greater trust and openness from my patients. I know where they're coming from—their passion, their mentality, their craziness. I understand what it is to be addicted to dancing—I've been there. The advantage to working with this patient population is that they are very much in touch with their bodies. They can help you get right to the root of the pain or the movement dysfunction. The musical companies we're under contract to—as well as the insurance companies—have come to realize that we save them money by keeping dancers working.

I've got to look out for my fellow dancers—they're family. If a company has been good to us, we'll keep working with them for free when their audiences get thin and they can't afford our services. But doing that isn't out of the ordinary for us. I feel that if you are practicing in the area of performing arts, you've got to love it, because it sure isn't going to make you rich.

PHYSICAL THERAPIST ASSISTANT

PREREQUISITES

Physical therapist assistants need many of the same skills and personality traits of the physical therapists who supervise them. They need fully as much physical stamina, for example. And they should both genuinely like and understand people, and be able to establish positive personal relationships with a minimum of difficulty.

PREPARATION

An associate's degree from an accredited physical therapy assistant program is required, either from a vocational-technical school, a junior or community college, or a university. In high school, those interested in becoming a physical therapist assistant should take courses in health, biology, mathematics, and computer skills. Forty-one states require that physical therapist assistants be licensed. Conditions for license renewal vary by state.

PRINCIPAL DUTIES

Physical therapist assistants work under the direct supervision of one or more physical therapists. They train patients in exercises, and carry out treatments developed by physical therapists at the direction of a physician. They assist in carrying out tests, evaluations, and more complex procedures; they observe and report patients' progress; and they administer heat, cold, electrical stimulation or ultrasound therapy at the request of the physical therapist.

OUTLOOK

The outlook for future employment of physical therapist assistants is even better than it is for physical therapists themselves, as the Department of Labor statistics on page 14 document.

EARNINGS

First-year physical therapist assistants can expect to earn approximately $22,500 annually. Those with several years experience can earn $26,000 or more per year.

    Resource: **American Physical Therapy Association**
                          1111 N. Fairfax Street
                          Alexandria, VA 22314

OCCUPATIONAL THERAPIST

Occupational therapists have a wider range of responsibilities than do physical therapists, in that their goal is to help patients lead independent, productive, and satisfying lives physically, mentally, and emotionally. They help patients not only to improve basic motor functions and reasoning abilities but also to compensate for permanent loss of function. In general, physical therapists concentrate on gross motor (large muscle) functioning; occupational therapists concentrate on fine motor (except for the hands) functioning. Occupational therapists use activities of all kinds ranging from computer-based exercises to caring for daily needs.

PREREQUISITES

Patience is needed to inspire trust and respect. Ingenuity and imagination in adapting activities to individual needs are desirable attributes. The job can be tiring, because occupational therapists are on their feet much of the time.

PREPARATION

A bachelor's degree in occupational therapy is the minimal requirement for entry into this field. Also, 39 states require a license to practice occupational therapy. License applicants must have a degree or a post-bachelor's certificate from an accredited program, and pass a national certification exam given by the American Occupational Therapy Certification Board. Those who pass become registered occupational therapists. High school students interested in a career in occupational therapy should take courses in chemistry, biology, health, art, and the social sciences. Volunteer or paid experience in a related healthcare profession also is helpful.

Occupational Therapy Network

The American Occupational Therapy Association (AOTA) began offering an online information service, Reliable Source, to its members in 1994. The online conference and electronic mail services facilitate quick communication among members and with AOTA staff. Reliable Source also includes a bibliographic database for occupational therapy literature with more than 20,000 citations. Access to Reliable Source, through a personal computer and modem, is available through an annual subscription.

PRINCIPAL DUTIES

Occupational therapists work in hospitals, clinics, rehabilitation facilities, long-term care facilities, extended care facilities, schools, camps, and patients' homes. For patients with permanent functional disabilities, such as spinal cord injuries or cerebral palsy, therapists may design and construct special equipment needed at home or at work. They develop and teach patients to operate computer-aided adaptive equipment, such as microprocessing devices that aid walking, communicating, or operating telephones and television sets. "Industrial therapists" help the patient find and hold a job, arrange employment, plan work activities, and evaluate the patient's progress.

In schools, occupational therapists evaluate children's fine motor abilities, recommend therapy, modify classroom equipment, and in general help children participate as fully as possible in school programs and activities.

Recording patients' activities and progress is an important part of an occupational therapist's job. Accurate records are essential for evaluating patients, billing, and reporting to physicians.

OUTLOOK

Employment of occupational therapists is expected to increase much faster than the average for all occupations through the year 2005 due to anticipated growth in demand for rehabilitation and long-term services. Medical technology that makes it possible for more patients with critical problems to survive will increase the need for occupational therapy for the survivors. Also, an increased population of those over seventy-five years of age will similarly translate to an increased need to provide therapy for age-related disabilities.

EARNINGS

The average occupational therapist entry-level salary is a little below $40,000. Experienced occupational therapists earn between $45,000 and $50,000, on average.

Resources: **Education Department**
American Occupational Therapy Association
4720 Montgomery Lane
Bethesda, MD 20824

Director, Accreditation Department
American Occupational Therapy Association
4720 Montgomery Lane
Bethesda, MD 20824

Green-Thumb Therapy

Gardening is an ideal hobby for people with back problems, muscle problems, weak vision, and other physical disorders. It may also be recommended to people confined to wheelchairs as long as the necessary adjustments in working tools and environment are made. (Therapeutic gardening tips can be obtained from the American Horticultural Therapy Association.)

OCCUPATIONAL THERAPIST ASSISTANT

PREREQUISITES

Similar to those for an occupational therapist.

PREPARATION

Occupational therapist assistant (OTA) programs are accredited by the American Occupational Therapy Association. Providing the applicant has a high school diploma, two educational routes are available: (1) a two-year associate's degree program offered by community colleges, and (2) a one-year, nondegree program offered by vocational and technical schools. Graduates of either type of program are eligible to take a certification exam leading to a COTA, or certified occupational therapist assistant, designation.

PRINCIPAL DUTIES

Occupational therapist assistants work under the supervision of occupational therapists and perform much of the routine work (often some of the more creative work, as well) dictated by the particular program being administered and the setting.

OUTLOOK

Employment opportunities for occupational therapist assistants are expected to grow much faster than the average for all occupations for the next several years.

EARNINGS

The average entry-level salary for occupational therapist assistants is just under $25,500. The annual salary for an OTA with several years' experience can exceed $30,000.

>Resources:	Education Department
American Occupational Therapy Association
4720 Montgomery Lane
Bethesda, MD 20824

>Director, Accreditation Department
American Occupational Therapy Association
4720 Montgomery Lane
Bethesda, MD 20824

CHAPTER 15
Pursuing Careers in Public Health

A large number of this nation's major healthcare problems handled by public health professionals involve broad-based social issues such as homelessness, infant mortality, substance abuse, child and spousal abuse, mental illness, violence, and the spread of sexually transmitted diseases such as HIV/AIDS and Hepatitis B. Public health professionals also help control the spread of airborne, waterborne, and food-borne diseases through research, community education, contact investigations, and on-site inspections. Public health professionals protect citizens from consuming contaminated food or water by regulating the employment of food service workers.

Here are a few of the statistics that motivate tens of thousands of men and women to pursue undergraduate and advanced degrees in public health each year, at one of 26 accredited schools of public health:

- More than 35 million Americans have neither health insurance nor access to adequate health care.
- The suicide rate for young American Indians is nearly twice that for white youths.
- An estimated one million Americans are infected with the HIV virus.
- Homicide is the leading cause of death among African-American youth.
- Diabetes is twice as prevalent for Hispanic-Americans aged 45–74 as it is for non-Hispanic Americans.
- During their first year of life, African-American infants are more than twice as likely to die as are white infants, largely because of lack of access to medical care.
- Most U.S. hazardous waste sites are near communities reporting a disproportionate share of toxic effects.
- Ten to fifteen million Americans are estimated to be infected with the germ that causes tuberculosis (TB).

By contributing their specialized knowledge, skills, and sensitivity, public health workers hope to change conditions such as these, and thus help break the cycle that continues to limit the potential of individual achievement and the future of our society.

PREREQUISITES

Although some graduate-level public health positions pay extremely well, most other jobs are supported by a combination of government grants and taxpayer money. For this reason salaries are often not competitive with those in private industry. Committed public health professionals achieve job satisfaction in other ways, however: through job diversity, for example; as well as the dynamic blend of social, economic, political, and medical challenges inherent in all public health positions.

Public Health: Past and Present

The U.S. Public Health Service originated in 1798 as a medical service for merchant seamen. The service expanded over the years, gradually adding public health functions, including research. But it was not until 1912 that it was given its current name to reflect this growing public health role.

Some hallmarks of progress since that time:

- Smallpox has been eradicated worldwide.
- Polio caused by wild virus has not been seen in the United States since 1991.
- Diseases such as Legionnaire's, toxic shock syndrome, and hantavirus pulmonary syndrome have emerged, and subsequently have been identified and treated.
- Cardiovascular deaths have declined dramatically, in part because of government campaigns warning of the dangers of cigarette smoking and in part because of its collaborative efforts in research, patient care, and public education on managing hypertension.
- Diabetes mellitus is under better control. Recent research has demonstrated that striking reductions in complications of type I diabetes are possible with effective management.

PREPARATION

With a few exceptions, schools of public health are graduate institutions that require a bachelor's degree for entry. (A few schools offer a baccalaureate degree in a limited number of areas. Graduates are qualified to enter the field as entry-level professionals.) All schools offer a Master of Public Health (MPH), and most offer a Master of Science (MS). Doctoral programs prepare graduates for teaching, research, and upper-level administrative positions.

Most schools offer one or more of the following forms of assistance for disadvantaged students:

- Fellowships, assistantships, traineeships
- Tutorial assistance
- Summer preparatory programs
- Counseling and support groups
- Mentor programs
- Health Careers Opportunity Programs
- Job placement assistance

- Summer internships

(Such assistance varies by school. Request information about specific programs from schools you intend to pursue seriously.)

Careers for which schools of public health offer preparation include:

- *Public Health Statistician.* Through the study of biostatistics, these workers study the incidence of a particular disease (polio, measles, or influenza, for example) and how such incidence varies with different age, ethnic, and socioeconomic groups, as well as with different localities. They design research projects and research techniques to answer questions concerning disease and health.
- *Epidemiologist.* They are experts in the study, distribution, and causes of epidemic diseases—tuberculosis, for example.
- *Environmental Health Officer.* They are concerned with the total environment: the air we breathe, the water we drink, the food we eat, the buildings we live and work in, the vehicles we travel in, and the places we visit for work and play. Environmental health officers investigate restaurants as sources of food- or waterborne diseases, such as Salmonella or the E. coli bacteria. They are also called in situations when animals are suspected of rabies. Related areas of interest include pollution of various kinds, the control or elimination of environmental health hazards, safety issues on the job and at home, and our mental and physical health.
- *Occupational Health Nurse.* Occupational health nurses work in factories or offices that employ large numbers of workers. Their field of occupational safety and health has as its goal minimizing sickness, injury, and maladjustments to work that may arise as a result of a worker's association with the work environment.
- *Health Educator.* Health educators work both with the community as a whole and with groups such as labor unions, civic organizations, and voluntary health and church groups. They plan health fairs, arrange discussion groups, and prepare printed materials—activities designed to heighten awareness of health hazards and help people change to healthier lifestyles through the more efficient use of health services and risk reduction behaviors.

A complete list of the ten areas of specialization can be found in the table that follows. For detailed information about the public health curriculum, as well as on specific career opportunities, write:

>Association of Schools of Public Health
>1015 Fifteenth Street NW, Suite 404
>Washington, DC 20005

Career Opportunities and Earnings Potential within 1 to 3 Years with a Graduate Degree in Public Health*

Career opportunities exist across all areas of specialization. The following denotes the highest frequency of opportunities in each area.

SPECIALIZATION	SALARY RANGE	ADMINISTRATION/ MANAGEMENT	EDUCATION	COMMUNITY PRACTICE	RESEARCH	POLICY
Public Health Practice/ Program Management	$26,125 – $64,750	E	E	E		
Biostatistics	$21,000 – $40,000	M	E	E	E	M
Biomedical and Laboratory Practice	$20,000 – $50,000	H	H	E	E	M
Environmental Health Sciences	$28,250 – $91,250	H	E	E	E	E
Epidemiology	$24,250 – $86,500	M	E	E	E	E
Health Education & Behavioral Sciences	$21,000 – $50,000	H	E	E	H	H
Health Services Administration	$23,500 – $102,500	E	H	E	H	H
International Public Health	$20,000 – $55,000	M	E	E	H	H
Nutrition	$20,000 – $45,000	E	E	E	H	H
Occupational Safety and Health	$26,000 – $80,000	M	E	E	H	H

Legend: M = Moderate Level of Opportunity; H = High Level of Opportunity; E = Extremely High Level of Opportunity

*Reprinted courtesy of Association of Schools of Public Health.

PRINCIPAL DUTIES

Public health professionals have a wide range of options to consider in applying their academic qualifications—regardless of their specialty field—in five general areas of opportunity:

1) **Community Practice:** *These public health professionals work with rural or inner city populations on such diverse issues as environmental pollution, teen suicide and homicide, long-term care for the aged, and immunization and care for the homeless through street outreach. Possible job settings include rural health clinics, crisis centers, HIV/AIDS task forces, substance abuse centers, and environmental agencies. Typical job titles include Biostatistician, County Health Department; Physician, Substance Abuse Rehabilitation Center; Counselor, Migrant Worker Clinic; Community Health Nurse, Cuban-American Health Center; and Public Health Nurse (or Manager), Public Health Department.*

CompuServe, an online service provider, offers the Public Health Forum for anyone involved or interested in the public health field. Members are invited to drop into the "Workers' Lounge" to seek or offer advice, or just let off steam. Following is a Workers' Lounge message posted by a Philadelphia physician specializing in adolescent medicine, with a practice devoted to teenagers. Her message, "End of a Bad Week," follows:

Friends,

It's been a bad week. All I want to do is crawl into bed and cry. My last patient is what did it to me. She was a 12-year-old who came to me for a physical examination. Her mother works next door at another hospital.

She started having sex at 10. Her sexual partners are over 20 because "she doesn't like the younger boys." She's been with about 12 or 13. She's lost count, but she doesn't feel like that is a lot of partners at all.

She doesn't use protection because she wants to get pregnant. She just "loves" babies because they are so cute. She has her baby names all picked out. When I mentioned not having sex, she rolled her eyes. When I talked about the pill, she changed the subject.

She plans to be a pediatrician but she gets Ds and Fs in school. She smokes a pack of cigarettes a day, and marijuana every other weekend. She also drinks beer occasionally.

She wants to kill her mother sometimes because she makes her mad. She feels that it is justified to kill people if they make you angry. She said that she would kill me if I made her angry.

I did the best I could during the 1.5 hours I spent with her. She seems to like me. I told her mother to bring her back to see me OFTEN so we can continue talking. They both left satisfied.

I'm left wondering what the hell is happening to this world.

Liana Clark, M.D.

---

2) *Administration/Management:* These workers manage culturally diverse and complex health services programs in urban or rural areas, dealing with the uninsured and underinsured, or with health risk assessment or occupational safety and health. Possible job settings include federal, state, or local government agencies, hospitals and clinics, research foundations, and environmental protection agencies. Typical job titles include Hospital Administrator; Director, Indian Health Services; Executive Director, Community Health Center; and Staff Administrator, Family Planning Clinic.

3) *Education:* These workers enlighten others about preventing diseases and disabilities that disproportionately affect disadvantaged populations, such as HIV/AIDS and other sexually transmitted diseases, drugs and alcohol abuse, maternal and child health issues, and social violence. Possible settings include colleges and universities, public and private secondary schools, voluntary health agencies, tribal organizations, and industry. Possible job titles are Executive Director, Sickle Cell Foundation; Teen Pregnancy Prevention Coordinator; Community Health Nurse, AIDS Education Training Center; and Counselor, HIV/AIDS Task Force.

4) *Research:* These public health professionals contribute to improving the health of the community through cutting-edge basic and applied research in malnutrition, infectious

diseases, women's health, cancer epidemiology, and identification of environmental hazards. Possible settings include schools of public health, departments of preventive medicine, universities and medical centers, and centers for disease prevention and control. Possible job titles include Analyst, Diabetes Control Program; Research Scientist, Infectious Diseases; Addiction Control Specialist; and Surveillance Officer, State Health Department.

5) **Policy:** *These public health professionals help create change by formulating, implementing, and evaluating public policy in family planning, disaster training, cultural and ethnic equality, and environmental legislation. Possible settings include congressional offices, regulatory agencies, law offices, federal and state agencies, and think tanks. Possible job titles: Lobbyist, Mexican-American Coalition for Health; Division Director, World Health Organization; Medicaid Commissioner; and Assistant State Health Officer.*

OUTLOOK AND EARNINGS

Specific opportunities in all areas of public health are excellent. According to recent U.S. Bureau of Labor Statistics estimates, less than half of one percent of all M.D.s currently are specializing in public health careers. Acute shortages exist for specialists in environmental health, nutrition, and epidemiology, with no change expected in the immediate future. The rapid increase in sexually transmitted diseases (including HIV/AIDS), the increase in diseases once thought to be conquered (such as tuberculosis), and the appearance of new diseases (such as those caused by the Ebola virus), have brought with them an acute need for qualified educators, administrators, researchers, and advocacy leadership—in this country as well as throughout the world. The career opportunities table on page 131, stakes out career and earnings potential in significant fields of public health specialization for all five of the opportunity areas described above.

Drug-Resistant TB Spreads

Washington Post, Feb. 14, 1996—According to an article published in Wednesday's *Journal of the American Medical Association,* a family of potentially fatal drug-resistant strains of tuberculosis that were first identified in New York in 1992 have spread to other cities in the United States and Europe. Researchers from the New York-based Public Health Research Institute who tracked the "W" strains of TB said that new drugs may be necessary to eliminate the bacteria, as the W strains do not respond to treatment with four of the most frequently used anti-TB medicines.

ANOTHER WAY TO GET THERE

In 1995, after 25 years of distinguished practice as an obstetrician/gynecologist, Dr. Lowell Marbry (not his real name) was at the top of his profession. He was respected by his patients as well as the community, and life seemed full and rewarding—both personally and professionally.

Then, to the surprise of family, friends, and patients, Dr. Marbry sold his share of the established Connecticut three-doctor, 20-employee clinic he had run for the previous 12 years, and enrolled in Yale University's School of Epidemiology and Public Health. Dr. Marbry explains his decision:

Why am I back in school at age fifty? I think it has more to do with change than anything else. My interests changed; my perceptions changed. But most of all, medicine itself changed, and I was trying to keep up with it.

As president and managing partner of my practice, I was making decisions for all of the people who worked for me. But I realized that my background was very limited. I hired an accountant, a lawyer, and a complete support system, and as a consequence I didn't know what was going on. I had no computer skills; I had no understanding of business and how it is organized today—except what I was able to pick up from the people around me, which is not the way you want to learn. I felt like a dinosaur.

It also bothered me intellectually. I was given a brain to use, and it seemed to me that I wasn't using it. Sure, I was doing good—I was helping people, making a difference in their lives. And that was important, but I began to realize that it was not enough.

I wasn't problem-solving anymore; I was just in a routine—an automaton. I mean, how many ways are women going to deliver? They will have either a vaginal birth or a cesarean section. And how many ways are there to do a pap smear? After you've mastered your craft there comes a time when work becomes just a numbing, crushing, routine.

Finally, it was keeping me awake nights. And I said to myself, if this is what it's all about, I don't want to do it any more. Most of all, I did not want to project this dissatisfaction onto my patients and become the cranky old doctor we've all heard so much about. You want to be "Dr. Welby," and not some miserable, unkind, unfeeling person. But there is really a risk of being numbed out, and I felt that coming on.

Well, last year I ran into a colleague who told me that a former classmate was coming to Yale as Dean of the School of Public Health. I called him—we hadn't seen each other since med school—just to say hello. I told him I was really burned out, and that I had stopped learning and really felt out of touch with what was around me, and was looking to do something else.

He told me that, given my interest in policy and the structure of the healthcare system, there was a program that could teach me health policy and how it was made, and eventually train me to be a physician/manager/policy maker. He said this involved clinical decision making, not treating the patient.

For example, not *doing* a pap smear, but deciding how often a pap smear is *appropriate*—evaluating the adequacy of the pap smear. And then dealing with the ramifications: What do the results mean? How many women are having pap smears—and why?

This is a very important area in medicine today, because it has tremendous implications for cost control and the kind of treatment patients will have. It involves telling the clinical person doing the treating—be it a doctor or a nurse-practitioner or a midwife—that guidelines are appropriate for treatment.

There's a tremendous interest in getting physicians to create these kinds of guidelines and policies, because physicians have been there; they have treated. You don't want nonphysicians creating policy without input from physicians. When that is the case you get the kind of policy that forces women who give birth to leave the hospital in one day. A physician who had delivered even one baby would realize that that is a very bad idea. This is a policy area I would be very interested in—probably in the ob/gyn area, because my knowledge in other areas is general and not specific. They need physicians with specific knowledge.

In our program here, of the 30-odd students who entered the policy management track, 12 are physicians—and that number is increasing every year. There are cardiologists, anesthesiologists, family practitioners, ophthalmologists—all of whom have been on the front lines treating and are now going back to impact the healthcare system.

So that's what I'm going to do when I graduate. But just think: I lived in this town and didn't even know such a program existed. If I hadn't called my old classmate to have coffee after finding out he was dean of the school, I still wouldn't know. I probably would have wound up instead being that cranky old physician.

CHAPTER 16

Pursuing Careers in Radiology

"I have discovered something interesting, but I do not know whether or not my observations are correct."

This remark to a friend was the only mention Wilhelm Roentgen made to anyone about his discovery of x-rays in 1895. When Professor Roentgen was sure enough about his achievement to break the news some weeks later, it electrified the world and changed medical diagnosis forever.

Today, just over a century later, the ability to "see bones on film" has evolved into a branch of medicine known as radiology: including tools that embrace organ scanning, ultrasound waves, and nuclear magnetic resonance aiding in the diagnosis of disease and—particularly in the case of cancer—its treatment as well.

RADIOLOGIST

The education of a radiologist can involve nine to eleven years of medical school, and a specialization either in diagnostic radiology or radiation oncology (the treatment of cancer with a variety of radiation techniques). An estimated 90 percent of physician radiologists are board certified, one of the highest percentages of all American Medical Association-recognized specialties. As more becomes known about various forms of cancer and more types of cancer become treatable, the need for qualified radiologists will continue to increase. According to 1994 American Medical Association surveys, radiologists were the highest paid of all physicians that year, either specialists or in general practice.

Resources: **American Society of Therapeutic Radiology & Oncology**
1891 Preston White Drive
Reston, VA 22091

Radiological Society of North America
2021 Spring Street, Suite 600
Oak Brook, IL 60521

ANOTHER WAY TO GET THERE

Janis Brown was thirty-five and a mother of two by the time she decided to go to medical school. By that time she had explored several careers. Here's how it all happened:

Studying microbiology at the University of North Carolina, Janis planned to work in a laboratory after graduation. "As the time approached, though," she says, "it seemed kind of mechanical and boring. Feeding blood samples into machines didn't sound that exciting. I wasn't quite sure what to do. So, I did a great big 180 and got a job as a flight attendant for Pan Am.

"It seemed like a fun thing to do—and my only opportunity to do it." She flew for four years, living in Miami, New York, San Francisco, and Chicago, before it got to be too much.

"Crazy schedules and never being home," says Janis of those days. "The reward was a free trip to Europe. Well, when you've already been there five times in the last month, it doesn't give you a big thrill anymore."

In the meantime, she got married. After quitting the airline she had a baby, and then went back into microbiology as a graduate student at Northeastern University. While there, she taught biology and chemistry at Quincy Junior College. She liked the students and enjoyed teaching, but the curriculum became monotonous after about three semesters. "Freshman chemistry never changes. It's easy, but once you prepare your lectures and notes, you can teach from the same material forever."

So Janis took a job with the Red Cross doing research on plasma immune globulins to develop vaccinations for chicken pox and other diseases. After a few years the future at that job looked dim too, although she enjoyed the research. She thought she could combine that with teaching by getting a doctorate.

With full support from her family, Janis entered medical school at Boston University in 1982 with an open mind about what kind of doctor to become. By the end of her second year, she had settled on radiology.

"One of the choices you make is primary care versus a specialty. As I got exposed to clinical medicine, I decided I probably didn't have the personality for primary care. In primary care you have a defined patient population: These are your patients, you take care of them, and they see specialists from time to time, but usually they come to you for ongoing care. Some people find that very rewarding. To me it's much more rewarding to confront a clinical problem: This is what I need to treat, I do it right now, do it well, I dictate my report, and that's it; I move on to something else."

Having finished her doctorate, Janis did post-graduate training and a four-year residency at the Yale School of Medicine. At that point she was hired as a member of the faculty, and is now an assistant professor. She does clinical work with patients at the hospital, teaches med students in class and residents in the hospital, and performs original research in radiology.

Of working in the hospital, which takes about 80 percent of her time, Janis says: "Radiologists do a lot more patient contact and hands-on procedures than 20 years ago. That's changed a lot. One of the things that attracted me to radiology is that it's very high-tech and very dynamic. We've had a technology explosion in recent years—ultrasound, CAT scans, MRI, surgery involving imaging guidance—there's always something new going on. This is all terrific stuff, but it's also gotten very expensive, so there's got to be more emphasis on talking to patients, examining them, and putting your hands on them, and ordering one test instead of six."

Research keeps Dr. Brown on the cutting edge, too. She's constantly working on new projects, writing several papers a year for medical journals, and teaching medical students and residents.

"Radiology is a very dynamic curriculum. There are new things happening all the time. What I teach now about ultrasound is very different already than what I taught even two or three years ago. You have to always keep up with what's new."

She's still a good teacher, too. In 1993, Dr. Brown was awarded the school's Teacher of the Year honors, voted by the staff residents of the hospital.

RADIATION THERAPIST

Radiation therapists use highly sophisticated equipment to treat various kinds of cancer. They beam x-rays, gamma rays, electrons, and other kinds of radiation at cancerous cells, while at the same time protecting adjacent normal cells from exposure and damage.

PREREQUISITES

Radiation therapists are on their feet for long periods of time, and often must be on call for evenings and weekends. They may have to lift or turn disabled patients. They are prone to emotional burnout as a result of seeing extremely ill or terminal patients on a daily basis.

PREPARATION

Those interested in a radiation therapy career may take a one- or two-year hospital-sponsored program leading to a certificate; a two-year associate's degree; or a four-year program leading to a bachelor's degree. The American Society of Radiologic Technologists, however, has set the year 2000 for requiring a bachelor's degree for entry into the profession. Successful completion of educational requirements entitles students to take a four-hour competency exam leading to certification. Approximately 25 states require radiation therapists to be licensed.

PRINCIPAL DUTIES

Radiation therapists must position patients under the equipment with absolute accuracy, to expose affected body parts only. They also check patients' reactions for radiation side effects, and give instructions and explanations to patients. Radiation therapists help to maintain equipment, and they assist in the preparation and handling of various radioactive materials used in procedures.

OUTLOOK

The employment of radiation therapists is expected to grow much faster than the average for all occupations for the next several years. Today there is a shortage in most parts of the country.

EARNINGS

Entry-level salaries for radiation therapists average about $25,000 annually. Experienced radiation therapists can earn between $30,000 and $37,000 on average.

Resources: American Society of Radiologic Technologists
15000 Central Avenue, SE
Albuquerque, NM 87123
(career and educational information)

American Registry of Radiologic Technologists
1255 Northland Drive
Mendota Heights, MN 55120
(certification information)

Radiology Celebrates 100 Years

At the 100th anniversary of Wilhelm Roentgen's discovery of x-rays, held in Chicago, radiology professionals both applauded their past and awaited their future. Among the presentations, here are a few that got the attendees' attention:

- A virtual reality technology to aid in diagnosing colon and lung cancer

- Magnetic resonance imaging-guided radiofrequency for destroying brain tumors
- MRI techniques for imaging the entire body in 18 seconds
- Some very post-mortem findings about Otzi, the Bronze Age "Ice Man"
- The unveiling of a downloadable cadaver, which warrants a bit more detail:

"The Visible Man" was created from thousands of images of a human body collected with state-of-the-art radiographic and photographic techniques. The Visible Man was generated from digitalized data compiled from the body of a thirty-nine-year-old man executed by lethal injection in Texas. The body was embedded in gelatin, frozen, and sliced axially into more than 1,800 sections 1 millimeter thick, using a laser-guided technique. As each cross-sectional slice was removed, a newly exposed surface was photographed.

Reconstruction of the data can be rotated in space, viewed in any plane, dissected, and reassembled. In the future, any anatomical part can be extracted from the body and viewed separately. Structures such as blood vessels can be followed throughout the body, and their relationship to other structures, such as organs and bones, can be seen.

There is no charge to access the Visible Man, but you will need a computer with 15 gigabytes of storage space, and up to two weeks of uninterrupted Internet time for downloading.

RADIOGRAPHER

Radiographers produce x-ray films of parts of the human body for use in diagnosing medical problems.

PREREQUISITES

Radiographers need an attention to detail, and the ability to communicate instructions clearly and precisely. Emotional stability and a genuine interest in helping people are definite assets.

PREPARATION

Radiographers must have a high school education for consideration. Many hospitals sponsor two-year accredited programs, as do many community and junior colleges, leading to an associate's degree. A number of programs leading to bachelor's degrees offer specific radiologic technology baccalaureates.

PRINCIPAL DUTIES

Radiographers prepare patients for radiologic examinations by explaining the procedure, and by positioning patients so that the correct parts of the body can be radiographed. They place the x-ray film under the part of the patient's body to be examined and make the exposure. They then remove the film and develop it.

Experienced radiographers may perform more complex imaging tests. For fluoroscopies, radiographers prepare a solution of contrast medium for the patient to drink, allowing the radiologist to see soft tissues in the body. Some radiographers operate computerized axial tomography (CAT) scanners to produce cross-sectional views of patients and are called CAT scan technologists. Others operate machines using giant magnets and radiowaves rather than radiation to create an image, and are called magnetic resonance imaging (MRI) technologists.

OUTLOOK

Employment of radiographers is expected to grow faster than the average for all other occupations over the next several years. This is likely to be more true of CAT scan and MRI technologists than for radiographers specializing in x-rays. The high cost of equipment is the single greatest inhibitor to a more extensive use of CAT scans and MRIs.

EARNINGS

Entry-level radiographers specializing in x-ray work earn an average of from $22,000 to $27,000 annually. Those specializing in CAT scan and MRI technology earn 10–15 percent more.

Resources: American Society of Radiologic Technologists
15000 Central Avenue, SE
Albuquerque, NM 87123
(career and educational information)

American Registry of Radiologic Technologists
1255 Northland Drive
Mendota, MN 55120
(certification information)

DIAGNOSTIC MEDICAL SONOGRAPHER

Diagnostic medical sonographers use equipment to send high-frequency sound waves into areas of the patient's body, which then create reflected echoes collected to form an image.

PREREQUISITES

Much the same as for radiation therapists.

PREPARATION

Educational programs for sonographers may be one, two, or four years in duration, depending on program design, objectives, and the degree or certificate awarded. Applicants to the one-year program must have qualifications in a clinically related allied health profession. Applicants to two-year programs must be high school graduates, with credits in basic science.

PRINCIPAL DUTIES

Sonographers project non-ionizing, high-frequency sound waves to form an image that is viewed on a screen. The image is either recorded on a printout strip or photographed for interpretation and diagnosis by physicians. Sonographers explain the procedure, record additional medical history, and then position the patient for testing. Sonographers look for subtle differences between healthy and pathological areas, and judge if the images are satisfactory for diagnostic purposes. Sonographers may specialize in neurosonography (brain), vascular sonography (blood flow), echocardiography (heart), abdominal sonography (liver, kidneys, spleen, and pancreas), obstetrical/gynecological sonography (female reproductive system), and ophthalmological sonography (eye).

OUTLOOK

The employment outlook for diagnostic medical sonography continues to exceed the supply, by some margin.

EARNINGS

According to 1995 Society of Diagnostic Medical Sonographers figures, the annual salary for sonographers with less than one year of experience is just under $30,000.

Resources: **Society of Diagnostic Medical Sonographers**
12770 Coit Road, Suite 508
Dallas, TX 75251
(career and curriculum information)

American Registry of Diagnostic Medical Sonographers
600 Jefferson Plaza, Suite 360
Rockville, MD 20852
(certification information)

NUCLEAR MEDICINE TECHNOLOGIST

Nuclear medicine combines radioactivity with chemistry, physics, mathematics, computer technology, and medicine to diagnose and treat disease. Nuclear medicine can provide information about both the structure and function of virtually every major organ system within the body.

PREREQUISITES

Skill sets and personality traits for nuclear medicine technologists are much the same as those for radiation therapists.

PREPARATION

Nuclear medicine technology programs range in length from one to four years and lead to a certificate, associate's degree, or bachelor's degree. One-year certificate programs are for healthcare professionals only, especially radiologic technologists and ultrasound technologists wishing to specialize in nuclear medicine. They also attract medical technologists, registered nurses, and others who intend to change fields or specialize. About half of all states require technologists to be licensed. In addition, all nuclear medicine technologists must meet the minimum federal standards on the administration of radioactive drugs and the operation of radiation detection equipment. More than 100 accredited nuclear medicine technology programs currently offer instruction and clinical internship.

PRINCIPAL DUTIES

Nuclear medicine technologists: (1) prepare and administer radioactive chemical compounds, known as radiopharmaceuticals; (2) perform patient imaging procedures using sophisticated radiation detecting instrumentation; (3) accomplish computer processing and image enhancement; (4) analyze biologic specimens in the laboratory; and (5) provide images, data analysis, and patient information to the physician for diagnostic interpretation. Possible career avenues for nuclear medicine technologists include research and development, education, administration, industry sales, and technical consulting.

OUTLOOK

Employment of nuclear medicine technologists is expected to grow much faster than the average for all occupations for the next several years. One factor will be the expanding clinical use of positron emission tomography (PET), which provides a new means of studying biochemistry and metabolism within living tissues.

EARNINGS

Typical entry-level salaries range from $20,000 to $32,000 per year, with the average just under $29,000.

Resources: Society of Nuclear Medicine—Technologist Section
1850 Samuel Morse Drive
Reston, VA 22090
(career and curriculum information)

Nuclear Medicine Technology Certification Board
2970 Clairmont Road, NE, Suite 610
Atlanta, GA 30329
(certification/registration information)

CHAPTER 17

Pursuing Careers in Veterinary Medicine

Veterinarians care for pets, livestock, and sporting and laboratory animals. They also protect humans against diseases carried by animals. A number of veterinarians engage in research, food safety inspection, or education. Some work with physicians and scientists on research or to prevent and treat diseases in humans. Veterinarians also practice in regulatory medicine or public health.

Veterinarians help prevent the outbreak and spread of animal diseases, and perform autopsies on diseased animals. Rabies, for example, can be transmitted to humans. Some veterinarians specialize in epidemiology or animal pathology. They control diseases transmitted through food animals, or deal with problems of residues from herbicides, pesticides, and antibiotics in animals used for food.

VETERINARIAN

PREREQUISITES

Veterinarians must be good decision makers, especially in emergencies. They should have keen powers of observation. (Their patients can't tell them where it hurts or what other symptoms they may have.) Veterinarians should be able to calm animals that are upset, and get along with animal owners. They also need good manual dexterity. Veterinarians who are self-employed must have all of the necessary small-business-owner skills. Competition for veterinary school is intense; a high grade point average is essential.

PREPARATION

Every state requires that veterinarians be licensed. To obtain a license, applicants must have a Doctor of Veterinary Medicine (D.V.M or V.M.D.) degree from an accredited school, and pass a state board examination. Veterinarians who seek specialty certification in one of the 20 areas available to them (ophthalmology, pathology, or surgery, for example) must complete a two- to five-year residency program and pass an examination.

A D.V.M. degree requires a minimum of six years of college, consisting of at least two years of preveterinary study. Most applicants to veterinary programs have completed four years of college. Training includes clinical experience in diagnosing and treating animal diseases, performing surgery, and laboratory work in anatomy, biochemistry, and other scientific and medical subjects. (For positions in education or research, a master's or Ph.D. degree usually is required, in addition to a D.V.M.) Twenty-seven schools are accredited by the Council on Education of the American Veterinary Medical Association, in 26 states.

PRINCIPAL DUTIES

Veterinarians diagnose medical problems, dress wounds, set broken bones, perform surgery, prescribe and administer medicines, and vaccinate animals against diseases. They also advise owners on care and breeding. Some veterinarians care for zoo or aquarium animals or for laboratory animals.

Veterinarians usually treat pets in hospitals and clinics. Those in large animal practice usually work out of well-equipped mobile clinics and may drive considerable distances to farms and ranches. They may work outdoors in all kinds of weather. Veterinarians can be exposed to disease and infection and may be kicked, bitten, or scratched.

OUTLOOK

More than 50,000 veterinarians practice today in the United States, about one third of them self-employed in solo or group practices. Employment of veterinarians is expected to grow about as fast as the average for all occupations over the next several years. The outlook is particularly good for veterinarians with specialty training. Demand for specialists in toxicology, laboratory medicine, and pathology is expected to increase.

EARNINGS

The average starting salary for veterinary medical college graduates (most veterinarians do not perform internships or residencies) is just over $30,000, with a range from $25,400 to $33,300. The average income of veterinarians in private practice is just over $63,000, and owners of private clinical practices is just under $80,000. Owners of larger practices can earn well over $100,000.

Resource: American Veterinary Medical Association
1931 N. Meacham Road, Suite 100
Schaumburg, IL 60173

ANOTHER WAY TO GET THERE

After spending four years as a successful veterinarian, Dr. Stuart Leland is finishing up a three-year fellowship in laboratory animal medicine at the Yale School of Medicine. As he embarks on a new career phase, Dr. Leland reflects on the many choices that led him to this point.

It's a scary thing about the health profession—by the time you get where you're going you've got five to eight years of post-graduate education invested, and there's a great fear of changing careers. At the same time, there's so much flexibility within the medical field—whether it's basic or applied research, clinical medicine, administration, or counseling. With some retraining, one may easily head down a different yet related path.

The first time I applied to veterinary school, I failed to get in. At the time I was really starry-eyed about the whole idea of being a vet. As a result of a post-rejection interview offered by the school, I worked for a year in a couple of veterinary hospitals. It helped me to understand more clearly what I was getting into. The next time I applied I was accepted, and went to Cal-Davis.

In vet school I decided on an equine curriculum. I started working with small animals almost by accident, and ended up loving it. Small animals offered more diagnostic and therapeutic challenges than horses. With horses, you either work with valuable performance animals that are worth a tremendous amount of money or with backyard animals that people don't value enough to pay for good veterinary care.

Your first job out of vet school is very important—it can have a profound effect on the kind of medicine you practice the rest of your life. Unlike students of human medicine, most veterinarians do not perform internships or residencies. This means your first employer molds your medical and surgical skills. The problem for a lot of inexperienced veterinarians is they end up working in practice with an employer who does not practice state-of-the-art medicine. This means that bad habits are learned that can be difficult to change.

I was lucky in that regard, because my internship provided me with a sound foundation and the necessary confidence. The problem I had was that after about two years as an associate I realized I was not being challenged intellectually. I was not performing the diagnostic and therapeutic workups I had been trained to perform. Most people didn't have pet insurance, so the workup and therapeutic options were limited financially.

In veterinary school you get to do a lot of fancy tests, use fancy equipment; but in the real world many people simply cannot afford that stuff. So you deal with skin diseases and vaccinations most of the year. Lack of intellectual stimulation was a complaint many of my classmates were also experiencing. Vets work very hard, and burnout is well known in the profession. I worked every Saturday, and was on emergency call every other night. I met a lot of veterinary owners who were on a second marriage, or complained about never seeing their kids.

So I decided to try something different. I went into business as a relief vet, filling in when other vets were away or on vacation. I brought them a valuable service, and they were glad to pay a premium for it. The interesting thing was that I got to meet a lot of veterinarians, and I found considerable dissatisfaction in vets with 15 or 20 years' experience. I started thinking that maybe this wasn't what I wanted to do forever.

I became interested in laboratory animal medicine, and landed a postdoctoral fellowship at Yale. Fundamentally, lab animal veterinarians are involved with all aspects of research using animal models of human diseases. Initially, I had a number of ethical questions. Nobody wants to see mistreatment of animals, but the research is ultimately designed to benefit human lives.

Laboratory animal medicine involves administrative, medical, and research skills. As an administrator I am responsible for the management and organization of the facility. This includes ensuring compliance with all codes, laws, and regulations, from safety to building specs. As a clinician I am responsible for keeping diseases out of the colony, and properly diagnosing and treating problems. Finally, as a collaborator in the research field, I am responsible for helping to design, implement, teach, and assist in the most effective use of animals. There's tremendous potential in this field. With the advent of transgenic (inserting a new gene) and knockout (removing a gene) technology, current predictions are that the use of laboratory animals will increase.

My goal after this is an assistant professorship, though I feel both capable and marketable to pursue other career pathways. Ultimately, I see myself as director of laboratory facilities at a medical institution, a medical school, a VA hospital, a biotechnology company, or within the pharmaceutical industry.

I think having a veterinary background has been a great plus: I bring a different perspective to the research lab than people who are Ph.D.s and primarily investigators. It makes me a more useful team member.

I really enjoy what I do. It's not at all what I had in mind when I started out in animal science. There were many different options at each step, and now I feel it's all coming together in a useful and coherent manner. And I never had to start over at square one!

Pursuing Careers in Veterinary Medicine

VETERINARY TECHNICIAN

Veterinary technicians provide support and assistance to veterinary doctors. They work in whatever environment a veterinarian may be found: animal hospitals, kennels, clinics, zoos, and laboratories.

PREREQUISITES

Patience, compassion, and a willingness to be part of the animal healthcare team are important assets for a veterinary technician.

PREPARATION

Applicants for an accredited veterinary technician program need a high school diploma. Sixty-five such programs exist in 39 states, most of them two-year associate degree programs, but several four-year bachelor's programs are available as well. The core curriculum includes fundamentals of chemistry, applied mathematics, communication skills, humanities, and biological science.

Alternative Veterinary Medicine

Dr. Allen Schoen, D.V.M., carries Chinese herbal remedies and acupuncture needles in his black bag alongside syringes and stethoscope. "Ninety-five percent of what I do is alternative," says Dr. Schoen. "It's not that I don't believe in Western medicine. I just think we should look at every possible way to make animals heal."

The Sherman, Connecticut, veterinarian once used acupuncture needles to sedate a Danish stallion injured in a trailer accident. Moments after he massaged the animal's misaligned pelvis back into position, it awoke pain-free.

Schoen records this and other holistic successes in his book, *Love, Miracles and Animal Healing* (Simon & Schuster). The department of acupuncture he founded in 1982 at the Manhattan Animal Medical Center now has 80 members.

Years ago Schoen was called by colleagues "the vet of last resort," because of his ability to resurrect terminal patients. Now others can share his gift.

PRINCIPAL DUTIES

The veterinary technician is the person who performs much of the laboratory testing procedures. Lab assignments usually include taking and developing x-rays, peforming parasitology tests, and examining various samples taken from the animal's body, among them blood. In a clinic or private practice, a veterinary technician also assists the veterinarian with surgical procedures. This generally entails preparing the animal for surgery, administering and controlling anesthesia, tracking the surgical instruments, and monitoring vital signs.

Veterinary technicians also perform ear cleaning and nail clipping as part of regular animal care. In most settings, they record, maintain, and order pharmaceuticals, equipment, and supplies.

OUTLOOK

Veterinary technicians are in demand, and the outlook for employment is very good. The field is not affected adversely by the economy, and thus offers considerable stability.

EARNINGS

Average starting salaries for veterinary technicians range from $14,500 to $22,000. Average salaries for experienced technicians range from $16,000 to $27,000.

Resources:	**American Veterinary Medical Association**
1931 N. Meacham Road, Suite 100
Schaumburg, IL 60173
(career and educational information)

American Association for Laboratory Animal Science
70 Timber Creek Drive, Suite 5
Cordova, TN 93018
(certification information)

CHAPTER 18

Jobs Available to High School Grads

Perhaps some of you turned immediately to this chapter rather than slog through the first 17. If so, you probably had your reasons. Not everyone can afford to go to college, for one thing. The fact is, a college degree—or even an associate's degree—is not a condition for finding a job in healthcare. Many options offer a point of entry without post-secondary credentials. Almost all of the occupations described below require a high school diploma or equivalent. Working at one of them is a way to "try on" a career before making a commitment that could waste a great deal of time and money.

There are occupations available without a diploma in addition to those described in this chapter. Let's say physical therapy interests you, for example. If you read Chapter 14, you will see that a position as a therapy assistant or aide is one that a high school grad can apply for successfully. For this reason you may want to check out appropriate specialty areas.

So don't depend on this chapter alone to determine your healthcare career-search strategy. Here's a more assertive way:

1) *Pick a career that interests you.*
2) *Read the chapter in this book that describes it.*
3) *Identify an entry-level position that would take you a step closer to an informed career decision.*
4) *Determine appropriate job-search strategy with the tools described in Chapters 19, 20, and 21.*

Before executing your plan, however, you have two other chores to get you on the right track:

1) *Go to the library and read all you can about the occupation that interests you. If your library skills are weak, ask a librarian for help. (Many libraries have a "career corner" to assist people with job-search problems.)*
2) *Talk to professionals in the career area you have selected, to assure yourself both that the information you have about it is accurate and that you have enough data to make an intelligent decision. (Information interviewing is covered more thoroughly in Chapter 20; see also Appendix D.)*

The number after each job description that follows indicates the growth quotient (G.Q.) for this occupation over the next several years. Only those occupations are listed that are expected to grow at either the same rate or faster than all other occupations over the next several years, as determined by U.S. Department of Labor analyses. The growth-rate codes for the alphabetically listed occupation titles below are as follows:

G.Q.-1—Much faster than all other occupations

G.Q.-2—Faster than all other occupations

G.Q.-3—As fast as all other occupations

ANIMAL ATTENDANT *(G.Q.-2)*

Advertisements for this position may also be listed under "animal groomer" or "kennel attendant." Animal attendants are trained on the job; there are no formal education requirements. Much of the work is physically demanding and can be unpleasant. (Somebody has to clean out those cages, and nobody is lower on the pecking order than the kennel attendant.) The advantage is that you will get a chance to observe veterinary technicians and technologists in action, be able to ask them and the veterinarian(s) any questions you have, and make a general determination as to whether the field is for you. In small practices, this position can also include receptionist and veterinary technician assistance duties. Animal groomers and kennel attendants earn between $250 and $350 per week.

    Resource: **National Dog Groomers Association of America**
                          Box 101
                          Clark, PA 16113

DENTAL ASSISTANT *(G.Q.-2)*

More than 200,000 dental assistants are employed by general dentists. Dental assistants work at chairside as dentists examine and treat patients. They prepare patients for treatment, hand dentists instruments, and keep patients' mouths clear by using suction and other devices. They also type records and do other office work. Dental specialists such as orthodontists and oral and maxillofacial surgeons employ dental assistants as well.

Dental assistants work in a very stable environment. As of 1994, those surveyed had been in their current jobs for an average of five years. Some dental assistants train to be dental hygienists. Others go into sales with dental supply companies, or become office managers in larger practices. The national average wage for a dental assistant is about $10 per hour, usually plus health insurance, vacations, and other benefits.

    Resource: **American Dental Assistants Association**
                          203 N. LaSalle
                          Chicago, IL 60601

DIALYSIS TECHNICIAN (G.Q.-2)

A technician's responsibilities vary from one dialysis unit to another. They may be limited to technical procedures and direct patient care, or they may include biochemical analyses, observations, and research studies. Although the number of formal training programs in two-year colleges or vocational schools is increasing, most programs are conducted informally in high schools with only a diploma necessary for qualification. Those students having the best opportunity will have taken biology, chemistry, mathematics, and health-related subjects. Training as a nursing assistant or emergency medical technician also will provide excellent preparation. Some hospitals offer paid training as a dialysis technician. Ask for a tour of a local dialysis center to test your interest and ask introductory questions. Dialysis technicians earn salaries of from $15,000 to $30,000 per year.

Resource: National Association of Nephrology Technologists
P.O. Box 4488
Bryan, TX 77805

DISPENSING OPTICIAN TRAINEE (G.Q.-2)

A number of employers hire people with no background in opticianry for informal on-the-job training or, in the case of larger providers, more formal apprenticeship. In the 21 states that license opticians, people without a college background train from two to four years as apprentices. High school courses in physics, algebra, geometry, and mechanical drawing are particularly valuable, because opticians use precision measuring instruments and other machinery and tools. Apprentices not only receive technical training but are taught office management and sales, as well. Beginning apprentices can expect to earn from $13,000 to $15,000.

Resource: Opticians Association of America
10341 Democracy Lane
Fairfax, VA 22030

EEG TECHNOLOGIST TRAINEE (G.Q.-1)

Electroencephalograph (EEG) technologists use an EEG machine to record brain waves as a first step toward diagnosing such diseases as brain tumors, strokes, and epilepsy. EEG technologists generally learn their skills on the job, although some complete formal training programs. Postsecondary training is offered in both hospitals and community colleges. Technologists should have manual dexterity, good vision, writing skills, and an aptitude for working with electronic equipment. Applicants with a bent toward science and who have taken high school courses in chemistry, physics, and advanced mathematics will stand the best chance for success. EEG technologists in large hospitals can advance to jobs performing more difficult tests and then to chief EEG technologist (also usually the laboratory manager). The average minimum annual salary of an EEG technologist is about $20,000.

> Resource: American Society of Electroneurodiagnostic Technologists, Inc.
> 204 W. Seventh Street
> Carroll, IA 51401

EKG TECHNICIAN TRAINEE *(G.Q.-3)*

One-year certificate programs still exist for EKG technicians, but most are still trained on the job by an EKG supervisor or cardiologist. On-the-job training usually lasts from eight to sixteen weeks. Those looked at most seriously to become trainees are often people already in the healthcare field, such as nursing aides. Electrocardiograph technicians (the long name) take "basic" EKGs by attaching electrodes to a patients's chest, arms, and legs, and then manipulating switches on the electrocardiograph machine to obtain the reading. The test is done before most kinds of surgery and as part of a routine physical examination for people who have passed "middle age."

Although the employment of EKG technicians is expected to decline eventually, employment of cardiology technologists as a whole is expected to grow faster than average for all occupations. It is important to use this opening primarily as a stepping stone for more demanding and responsible technological positions in the cardiovascular field. Check the market situation in your area before committing to an apprenticeship. The median annual salary for EKG technicians is about $17,500. The average salary for cardiovascular technologists (the next level up), however, is about $29,000.

> Resource: American Society for Cardiovascular Professionals
> 10500 Wakeman Drive
> Fredericksburg, VA 22407

EMERGENCY MEDICAL TECHNICIAN *(G.Q.-2)*

Emergency medical technicians (EMTs) offer on-scene care to victims of automobile accidents, heart attacks, near drownings, gunshot wounds, and other medical emergencies. Following instructions from a dispatcher, EMTs drive specially equipped emergency vehicles to the site of emergencies. When necessary, they request additional assistance from police, fire, or electric company personnel. They are responsible for the initial assessment, stabilization, and transportation of an injured or medically ill person. All EMTs attend a basic 120-hour training program. There are four levels of EMT:

1) ***Medical Response Technician (MRT):*** *The level attained by most fire fighters and some police officers to provide emergency assistance before medical or paramedical treatment is available*

2) ***EMT-Basic:*** *Staffs ambulances providing basic life support skills; may restore breathing, control bleeding, treat for shock, administer oxygen, bandage wounds, and assist heart attack victims*

3) ***EMT-Intermediate:*** *Undergoes an additional 65–80 hours of training; can perform such additional procedures as administering intravenous fluids and using defibrillators to give lifesaving shocks to a stopped heart*

4) ***EMT-Paramedic:*** *Provides extensive pre-hospital care; may also administer drugs orally and intravenously, interpret EKGs, and use complex equipment; undergoes an additional 600–1,000 hours of instruction, including clinical and field internships*

Because EMTs are employed by commercial firms, hospitals, municipal agencies, and fire departments, pay scales vary widely, from the mid-teens to the high thirties and above for qualified EMT paramedics. Make inquiries in your city or metropolitan area.

Resource: **National Association of Emergency Medical Technicians**
102 W. Leake Street
Clinton, MS 39056

HOME HEALTH AIDE *(G.Q.-1)*

Home health aides (also known as personal care attendants) help elderly, disabled, and ill people to live in their own homes instead of in a health facility. Successful home health aides like to help people and don't mind hard work. They also require a sense of responsibility, compassion, emotional stability, and a cheerful disposition. The National Home Caring Council requires 60 hours of training. Programs are offered by community colleges, adult education programs, and private agencies. Twenty states require such formal training, and many others recommend it.

A November 1995 Department of Labor analysis listed home health aides as one of the two occupations expected to grow the fastest in the United States over the next several years—in any industry. An additional 250,000 jobs are expected to be created by the year 2005. Home health aides in some parts of the country are paid by the hour, with a range of from $5 to $11. Salaried aides earn between $11,000 and $17,000 annually, but can earn more, depending on the situation.

Resource: **Home Care Aide Association of America**
519 C Street NE, Stanton Park
Washington, DC 20002

ANOTHER WAY TO GET THERE

Karen Sherman is working as a personal care attendant while she figures out a way to go to nursing school. Her life seems to be on overload these days, though. She works, takes classes at night, and still must find time to care for her three young children. This juggling act accounts for every minute of the day, but it is a clear indication of Karen's firm commitment to her nursing career.

As a PCA (personal care attendant) I'm on my feet all the time. I do EKGs, catheterizations, vital signs, blood pressures, ADL (activities of daily living), assist my spinal cord patients, put patients on the passive motion machine with a cool pack, and get patients ready for bed at night.

I originally became a PCA because my husband was laid off as a result of company downsizing, and we needed health benefits. That was a scary time. Things were not good for engineers in the Northeast, and companies were folding right and left.

At the time I was a makeup artist and had my own business. It was doing quite well, actually. I had worked for Clinique for years, so I knew about makeup applications and the "tricks of the trade." I would go to a bride's house on her wedding day and do her makeup. As a present to her bridesmaids, the bride would pay me extra to do the bridesmaids' makeup, too. I wasn't trying to sell any products—I had no products to sell—just my skills. Then I would teach my clients the techniques I used.

My favorite part of the business was helping people who had been born with facial birthmarks or defects, and using makeup to give them a more "normal" appearance. Even though the business was doing well, I became uncomfortable with a career where looks were the major priority. In my personal life I had started to question a lot of things, including the way women are pressured to revolve their whole lives around "looking good."

Even then, becoming a nurse was in the back of my mind, where taking care of people and the way patients were treated was more important than appearance. So when my husband got laid off, I had to give up the business. But I had been headed in that direction, anyway. I took a two-week course to become a CNA (Certified Nurse Assistant) and then went to a rehabilitation hospital, where they trained me as a PCA. Even though my work is hard, I really do love it. I love working with the elderly, and I've gotten to know some really nice people.

MEDICAL ASSISTANT *(G.Q.-1)*

Medical assistants (MAs) perform a variety of clerical and clinical duties. The clinical duties vary by state law, but often include taking medical histories, preparing patients for examination, collecting and preparing laboratory specimens, sterilizing medical instruments, and performing basic laboratory tests. In some states they are authorized to draw blood, prepare patients for x-rays, take electrocardiograms, remove sutures, and change dressings.

Experience can lead to specialized medical assistant jobs in podiatry, ophthalmology, medical technology; or advancement to office manager, medical records administration, phlebotomist, lab technology, and sometimes even to nursing school. Rapid growth is expected in all outpatient settings, where most medical assistant work is centered. For this reason, and also because of the rapid turnover (this is an excellent training ground for occupations with more responsibility), employment is expected to grow much faster than average as the health services industry expands. Compensation for medical assistants varies as widely as does the range of responsibilities. Factors include experience, skill level, and location. The average starting salary for graduates of accredited medical assistant programs is just over $15,000 annually, with an average for all MAs of just under $18,500.

Resource: American Association of Medical Assistants
20 N. Wacker Drive
Chicago, IL 60606

NURSING AIDE AND PSYCHIATRIC AIDE *(G.Q.-1)*

Nursing aides and psychiatric aides help care for physically or mentally ill, injured, disabled, or infirm individuals confined to hospitals, nursing or residential care facilities, and mental health settings. Nursing aides work under the supervision of nursing and medical staff. They answer patients' call bells, deliver messages, serve meals, make beds, and feed, dress, and bathe patients. They may also give massages, provide skin care, take temperatures, pulse, and blood pressure, and help patients get in and out of bed and walk.

Some employers (hospitals, clinics, nursing homes) do not require a high school diploma for nursing or psychiatric aide candidates, although many do. Also, some prospective employers are receptive to applications from middle-aged and older men and women. Ask about specific requirements at institutions of interest to you. Employment for both categories is expected to grow well ahead of the average for all occupations over the next several years, particularly for nursing aides.

Many hospitals are moving toward a higher-skilled worker than a nursing aide, combining the skills of a nursing aide and medical assistant, who can team with a nurse and provide more technical assistance than can a nursing aide alone. Nursing aides are likely to flourish in a nursing home environment, but less so in hospitals. Median annual earnings for nursing and psychiatric nursing aides working full-time are about $14,000. The lowest 10 percent earn about $10,000, and the highest 10 percent about $25,000.

Resources: **American Hospital Association**
Division of Nursing
840 North Lake Shore Drive
Chicago, IL 60611

American Health Care Association
1201 L Street NW
Washington, DC 20005

PART III
Job Search Strategies

CHAPTER 19

Creating a Master Résumé and Cover Letter

Now it's time to create the documents that will help generate interviews and job offers: your résumé and application letters. Sample curriculum vitae (C.V.) and résumés can be found on pages 177–255.

The résumé is a multi-purpose tool, crucial to your job search. Here are the roles a good résumé should play:

- Act as an advance communicator that lets employers know you are available
- Serve as a professional brochure, to be distributed among prospective colleagues for reference and evaluation
- Transmit your sense of self to a prospective employer through its content, form, and style
- Provide a current record of your professional accomplishments, skills, promotions, and career highlights

There is another important role a résumé plays, less tangible than those mentioned above but no less significant. The process of researching, developing, and refining one's most important professional accomplishments in an effective way can be a tremendous confidence builder.

With all of these important responsibilities, it is obvious that a résumé should be prepared with considerable care. Actually, it must be constructed or crafted rather than written. All its pieces must interlock with one another in seamless fashion, with meticulous attention paid to what has gone before and what lies ahead.

To reach this level of quality, be prepared to put together several drafts, working almost in the manner of a master chef reducing a multi-ingredient liquid to a fine sauce. "Omit needless words," wrote William Strunk in *The Elements of Style,* a classic primer on written communication still readily available. This is especially true for résumés.

One reason for this is that a resumé must communicate both totally and instantly. If you learn about a job opening from a classified ad or from the Internet, for example, there may be hundreds of other applicants. With this volume of response, company "first readers" (the executives or supervisors actually doing the hiring rarely go through all the resumés received) find themselves reading to *exclude* rather than *include* potential candidates.

If a hospital director of nursing needs to hire a new nurse supervisor for the operating room, for example, she may specify five essentials she wants her readers in the personnel department to look for in an applicant. If those qualities appear somewhere in the resumé but are not quickly identified, out goes the resumé. In such a situation, ten seconds may be as much time as an applicant has to make the first cut.

This means the various elements that a potential employer is looking for (upward mobility, tangible accomplishments, stability, and the like) must pop out and catch the reader's eye. You can accomplish this by the creative use of type and white space.

By underlining, using boldface or italics, or putting certain words or phrases in capital letters—all done in a systematic, consistent way, of course—different elements of a resumé can be made more visible. Similarly, by putting some "air" between entries, or spacing some kinds of data horizontally or vertically from others, all of the elements can be made easier to read, and more data can be taken in at a single reading. For example, two- to four-line entries are far easier to read than dense paragraphs of type, and are therefore far more likely to get read.

Omit Needless Words

"Vigorous writing is concise. A sentence should contain no unnecessary words, a paragraph no unnecessary sentences, for the same reason that a drawing should have no unnecessary lines and a machine no unnecessary parts. This requires not that the writer make all his sentences short, or that he avoid all detail and treat his subjects only in outline, but that every word tell."

—William Strunk, Jr.
The Elements of Style

ORGANIZING YOUR RESUMÉ OR C.V.

There are dozens of ways resumés can be written. Check your local bookstore and you'll find ten or more experts giving contradictory advice on the arcane art of resumé preparation. Some writers, in fact, advise not using resumés at all. The advice here is based on a survey of corporate executives and hospital human-resource directors, subsequently used by a New York career-counseling firm to guide their clients in resumé construction. The interviewers themselves were interviewed. Here is a capsulized version of the survey results, broken down into three categories: content, clarity, and style.

CONTENT
- Be sure the reader of your résumé can identify both your immediate objective and a summary of your job-related qualifications.
- Describe your accomplishments for each job in quantitative terms where possible, as well as the specific nature of each job.
- Organize your résumé in such a way that your professional level is clearly evident. If you have more than three years of job experience, for example, the "Education" section should come at the end of your résumé.
- Load the résumé in favor of accomplishments, skill, and responsibilities that pertain specifically to the job you are seeking. Eliminate excessive personal data and overly detailed descriptions of previous jobs.
- Be truthful about problem areas such as employment gaps and perceived job-hopping, but avoid including gratuitous information that may damage you.
- Always include career-related volunteer experience.

CLARITY
- For easier reading, limit job and accomplishment descriptions to four lines.
- Clearly and specifically state your position objective and summary of experience.
- Double-check to eliminate errors or inconsistencies in grammar or punctuation. If necessary, ask an English teacher or local newspaper editor for help.
- Be sure to clearly label all personal data (name, address, phone, e-mail, and FAX numbers).
- State your job history in reverse chronological order, making sure that multiple positions for the same company are not mistaken for individual employers.

APPEARANCE
- Invest in a quality typing and printing job.
- Choose paper of good weight and quality, standard size, and conservative color. (Ask a friend whose taste you respect for advice if you need it.)
- Avoid attention-getting special effects (e.g., mixed type styles, brochure format, photographs).
- Limit your résumé to two pages.
- Keep the "look" of your résumé appropriate to the position you are seeking.
- Take any measures necessary to eliminate typographical errors. If necessary, pay an expert for a final check.

CHRONOLOGICAL AND FUNCTIONAL RÉSUMÉ FORMATS

There are basically only two types of résumés: chronological and functional. If you decide to go to a professional résumé writer, or if résumé writing is included in any career counseling you contract for, you should know how to recognize these two basic types and be aware of the advantages and disadvantages of each. The chronological résumé is structured job by job, company by company. It begins with the present and works backward in time, with all accomplishments and skills tied closely to specific employers and positions. In the functional résumé, on the other hand, similar accomplishments and skills are grouped together regardless of employer in a one-page (or less) professional profile. (See pages 235 and 238 for examples.) A short job history usually follows, but it generally includes only the names of the institutions, job titles, and the time spent with each employer.

For all its good intentions, the functional résumé has one basic problem: It appears to be hiding something. Why is the applicant trying to avoid any association of jobs and duties, companies, and accomplishments? The perception, right or wrong, is that a functional résumé is being used to mask lateral or descending career moves, career changes, or job hopping.

If the perception is accurate, then a résumé is probably the wrong tool anyway. If the perception is inaccurate and there is nothing to hide, then a functional résumé will serve you badly.

TARGETING

Good writers write for specific audiences. As a résumé writer, your audience will depend on how widely you are casting your net. And if you intend to change jobs in terms of specialty or function, as well as consider positions in the specialty and function you just left, you will need to think about preparing a second or even a third résumé rather than write a single résumé in terms so general as to appeal to all possible employers.

No matter whom you are writing for, however, the point is to address your reader's specific needs. To do this you have to be able to communicate three essential levels of information:

1) *Knowledge of specialty*
2) *Knowledge of prospective employer*
3) *Knowledge of position or function*

Those of you writing your first résumés should emphasize how comprehensive and relevant your education is to the opportunity you are seeking. Include any summer, part-time, or volunteer jobs you have held, giving most space and attention, obviously, to those in the healthcare industry.

1) *If your goal is to re-enter the marketplace at or above the position you just left, you'll need to demonstrate your awareness of industry trends, problems, and promise, including any state-of-the-art responsibilities you have had or accomplishments you have attained.*
2) *Your knowledge of the prospective employer usually can be demonstrated in terms of the institution you just left. After all, if you are changing very little in terms of your career, a number of similarities will exist between your current employer and your next*

one. Your knowledge of other hospitals or clinics, for example, can be handled in the cover letters that accompany the résumés you send to those target employers. (In Chapters 20 and 21 you will learn more about researching target employers.)

3) *If you are moving up a notch, the position you are interested in probably will entail a job very much like the one your direct supervisor holds. Make sure your prospective boss can see which of your old boss's responsibilities you have handled or could handle. Those of you changing functions will find it tougher.*

Putting together the best possible résumé requires that you assemble all the professional, personal, and educational data that are relevant. This brings us to the components of the résumé itself.

RESUMÉ COMPONENTS

Objective

After identifying yourself by name, address, phone and FAX number, and e-mail address, describe the specific job you want. This entry, called the "Objective," along with the "Summary" section that follows it, sets the tone and positioning for the entire résumé. These sections will provide a perspective for every word that follows.

It is best if you can describe your ideal position in a single title. Examples are:

OBJECTIVE: Neonatal Nurse Clinician
OBJECTIVE: Social Worker/Case Manager
OBJECTIVE: Pharmacist
OBJECTIVE: Exercise Therapist

You may want to be even more specific, depending on your specialty or focus. For example:

OBJECTIVE: CARDIOLOGY NURSE—Cardiology research position with direct patient/physician contact

Write your objective broadly enough to encompass your desired position even if the job title changes from employer to employer, but stay as focused as possible to permit your reader to see where you are going. Do not generalize to appeal to a wider range of possibilities; just write additional résumés to reflect different opportunities you are considering.

If you spot an opportunity slightly at odds with your current objective but thoroughly consistent with your background, adjust your objective to match it. Suppose the cardiology nurse with the objective stated above learns about a staff position calling for ambulatory care experience. She has done that, so she simply changes enough of her objective to bring it in line with the job description:

OBJECTIVE: STAFF NURSE—Ambulatory care position with potential for administration or management

Or, suppose she sees another opening—again, not varying greatly from previous jobs she has heard about but slightly different from her objective of cardiology nurse in research. It might be reflected by a change in her objective as follows:

OBJECTIVE: CARDIOLOGY NURSE—Staff position with potential for administration or management

These differences may seem minor, but objectives set the tone for the way résumés are read. If you can reword your objective to reflect the precise nature of the job offered—legitimately reflecting your experience—you enhance your chances of getting an interview. And this may be the edge you need.

Summary

While the objective tells the reader exactly what it is you want to do, the "Summary," or "Career Highlights" section, tells in very specific terms why you are qualified to do it. The summary should distill your professional experience down to three to six power sentences that emphasize your skills, accomplishments, and any special qualifications you may have for the objective written just above it.

The summary is your opportunity to pull out all the stops. An accomplishment you are extremely proud of but that took place three jobs ago, for example, can and should be mentioned in this section. On a "traditional" résumé, the accomplishment would appear in the middle of page two and might never get read, especially if your résumé is being given a quick scan by a first reader.

Let's go back to the cardiac nurse's résumé:

SUMMARY: Experienced cardiac nurse in both staff and research situations. Skilled supervisor, leader, problem solver; ability to interact well with doctors, patients, and staff. Administrative background in budget analysis, scheduling, and admissions. Assertive, creative, and versatile.

Every word in her summary is position-specific, intended to match her credentials with the responsibilities of the job. The sole purpose of this careful matching is to improve the odds for a job interview. The summary is your best advance sales tool, so make the most of it.

On Writing Well

"Writing is hard work. A clear sentence is no accident. Very few sentences come out right the first time, or even the third time. Remember this as a consolation in moments of despair. If you find that writing is hard, it is because it *is* hard. It's one of the hardest things that people can do."

—William Zinsser
On Writing Well

To construct your summary, review your career to date and list all of the responsibilities, achievements, and skills you believe will qualify you for your next position. Eliminate or combine any major overlaps, and begin to group your qualifications by category.

FORMULATING YOUR OBJECTIVE AND SUMMARY

Those of you contemplating a slight career change should remember that the language you use in your résumé is as important as the message you are trying to convey. If the terminology of your old career is different from that of your new one, discard it. Prospective employers usually are unable to see the crossover value in skills and achievements attained in another industry or function. Therefore, if you are seeking a healthcare industry position and all of your experience is outside the industry, avoid the inside language of your previous industry and use terms a prospective employer will be comfortable with. Talk with a few people in the healthcare specialty you are entering, and show them your résumé draft to be sure your vocabulary is on target.

Look at those résumés beginning on page 196 that include objective and summary sections, and then use the the following form to help put together an effective objective and summary:*

OBJECTIVE

The objective should mirror the position you're after, either by specific title or by a brief generic description. Write your objective here:

....
....
....

Look at your objective to make sure it will be absolutely clear to the reader. What are the principal duties required for the position listed in your objective?

1. ....
2. ....
3. ....
4. ....

What abilities or skills will be needed for someone to be successful in the position listed in your objective?

1. ....
2. ....
3. ....
4. ....

---

* Forms used in this chapter are adapted from *Job Bridge,* © Wilson McLeran, Inc., New Haven, CT 06511.

SUMMARY

The objective states what job you're after; the summary tells why you're qualified to do it. Complete the following form to help you write your summary. In terms of the type of position you are seeking, what significant accomplishments highlighted your last two or three positions?

Position #1: (most recent)
Title:..

Overall Duties:
1..
2..
3..
4..

Significant Achievements:
What did you do?...
....
....
What were the results?..
....
....
What abilities or skills were required?.............................
....
....

(Repeat for positions before "Position #1.")

Now go back and circle those duties, accomplishments, and abilities that relate most closely to the position listed in your objective. Your goal is to make the best fit possible between the prospective job and your qualifications. So use only those accomplishments that relate specifically to the position you are seeking.

Using your circled items, write on a separate sheet of paper the summary of your qualifications for the position. (Refer to the sample résumés on pages 196–255 for models.) For maximum effectiveness, your summary should be no longer than four or five sentences.

Look at what you've written:
- Is it clear?
- Is it interesting?
- Are the ideas linked logically?

Write as many additional drafts as necessary to be satisfied with the result.

FORMULATING YOUR EXPERIENCE SECTION

The substance of any chronologically organized résumé is the description of specific jobs you've held for various employers. Many people think that a simple job description will suffice. Not so. More important by far is an indication of how well you performed in each position.

You should describe major responsibilities, of course, but concentrate even more heavily on the accomplishments you can legitimately claim as your own. This will give you a nucleus of information from which to frame a powerful, achievement-oriented "Experience" section. Use past achievements consistent with your present career direction, and spend as few words as possible on previous positions with no bearing on the kind of job you are after today. Similarly, devote more attention to current or recent career-related positions than on those held earlier in your professional life. Do not appear to be dwelling in the past. If you attained similar major goals early in your career as well as more recently, pack them in your current experience and keep the past relatively spare.

One exception to this advice is if you are in the process of returning to the healthcare industry after one or more years away from it. In this instance, the wiser course is to list first those early positions, responsibilities, and accomplishments on the résumé under a heading such as "Relevant Experience," and try to use the entire first page to chronicle this part of your professional background. That way your objective and summary will be followed by a description of the experience that most clearly backs up your intentions. The only possible drawback to this strategy is that employment dates for the job experience you are describing may go back a decade or more. Handle this with a footnote after the dates, such as "For current experience, see page 2."

Remember that your résumé will be important in your interview. Accomplishments should be broken up into bite-size pieces for the interviewer to spot and absorb quickly. You as the interviewee, on the other hand, should view each entry as the basis for a leading question, about which you have rehearsed responses of from ten seconds to ten minutes, determined by interviewer interest.

Think of your résumé as a script for both you and the interviewer. This is particularly true of the experience section. Each entry is a cue to be picked up by the interviewer as appropriate, and singled out for further questions if it piques interest or relates to the position available.

For that reason, it is extremely important not only to include your most impressive achievements but to list them in order of importance—almost the way you wrote a topic outline for an essay or composition in school. Where appropriate, quantify an accomplishment to further whet the reader's interest, and be sure to follow a main point with appropriate subpoints.

The cardiac nurse candidate whose objective and summary appeared earlier in the chapter is a good example of a slight career changer. After being let go from the consultant position she held with a cardiovascular equipment manufacturer after a company downsizing, she decided to go back to nursing. Her most recent experience is relevant because she demonstrated state-of-the-art equipment in her specialty to prospective customers on a day-to-day basis. Here is how she treated that experience:

- Wrote and presented educational seminars and inservices for physicians, staff and ancillary personnel in cardiac catheterization/angioplasty laboratory
- Maintained and increased knowledge base on current and new technologies by attending national and regional seminars
- Acted as consultant on product evaluations/introductions, during live-case and other areas of cardiology
- Maintained territory sales level (28 percent market share) for two five-month periods while sales position was vacant
- Successfully combined products and pricing strategies in response to wide variety of situational needs

Using a similar style, go back to the summary exercise that includes your job-by-job duties and accomplishments, and put them in final form for your experience section. (Consult the sample résumés on pages 178–255 as additional models.) The most important point to remember in writing and laying out this section is: Make all key aspects of every entry as clear and as visible as possible so that your reader will be able to take in your strengths at a single glance, and select for more careful reading those that relate closely to the target position. The layout of your résumé, in fact, is as important as its content.

The Right Word

"The difference between the right word and the almost right word is the difference between lightning and the lightning bug."

—Mark Twain

Miscellany

Here are a few personal opinions on whether you should include these frequently seen résumé entries:

Career-related hobbies—yes
Marital status, weight, height—no
State of health—no (it's always "excellent" anyway)
Photograph—no
"References available on request"—no (when they're needed, you'll be asked)
Military—career-related assignments only

PUTTING YOUR RÉSUMÉ ALL TOGETHER

Now you are ready to put your résumé together. Using the samples on pages 196–255 and the forms you have completed as models, write the first draft of your résumé on a separate piece of paper. Try to get your essential information on no more than two pages.
Hint: When writing your résumé, always think in terms of your objective.
- Write as many drafts as you feel are necessary to construct a finished product that pleases you.
- Ask your spouse and/or one or two colleagues to read your final draft and suggest additions, cuts, or changes.
- Have your résumé typed or typeset by a professional.

Résumés for the Internet

Those of you using Internet sources as part of your job search (see Chapter 20, pages 263–268) will prepare your résumés from a different perspective. Forget about paper quality, type size and face, and other visual elements considered earlier in this chapter. Many electronic job search services have their own fill-in-the-blanks form; others offer more spatial leeway. In either case, the burden of communication will be borne largely by the words you use.

In essence, the online and Internet job-search services act as your electronic executive recruiter, except that you do more of the work than you would with a recruiter. There is another similarity that works to your advantage. The physical appearance of a résumé is less important to a client working through a recruiter than, say, an employer you apply to directly. This means that the pressure is off regarding paper and type decisions. These will be made for you.

The control you *do* have over appearance has to do largely with spacing: Use white space to set you apart from the preponderance of type-dense résumés downloaded by employers. (You'll see several of each in the array of sample résumés that appear on pages 232–255.)

Curriculum Vitae

Although many physicians are comfortable with a standard résumé, most prefer a more detailed curriculum vitae (C.V.), particularly if they teach or write in addition to their clinical duties. (Some nurses applying for fellowships or research positions also find C.V.s more appropriate than a résumé.)

The biggest difference between a résumé and a C.V. is in "tone." Where a résumé is a selling tool without apology, a C.V. is more low-key. An assertive, accomplishment-laden summary section is out of place on a C.V. Most decisions to interview at the physician level are based on academic standing, board certifications, honors, awards, and publications. These speak for themselves and need no embellishment. (Sample C.V.s can be found on pages 178–194.) For detailed tips on preparing a C.V., as well as advice on the entire process of residency selection, see *Strolling Through the Match,* published by the American Academy of Family Physicians, 8880 Ward Parkway, Kansas City, MO 64114.

WRITING YOUR MASTER COVER LETTER

You will need a basic cover-letter format you can adapt for each of the situations that require a mailed résumé. Letters for any reason should never look as though they have been mass produced. If they do, it will guarantee that your résumé will see the bottom of a wastebasket before it gets read.

Here are the situations for which you'll want to develop cover letters:
- Responses to newspaper or trade journal ads
- Introductions to executive recruiters or employment agencies
- Applications to hospitals, HMOs or other institutions

Notice that the sample letters on pages 174 and 175 contain four elements, regardless of the situations for which they were written:

1) ***Attention.*** *It is essential to grab your reader immediately to assure that the rest of the letter gets read. This needn't be gimmicky; just state your business in as straightforward and powerful a way as you can. Rely on a news peg—perhaps a new development within your target institution (a major equipment purchase; a new hospital procedure) that triggered your letter in the first place.*

2) ***Interest.*** *In this section you'll need to describe in hard-hitting fashion the qualities you believe will merit the reader's attention. These qualities should fulfill the need specified in the attention paragraph.*

3) ***Conviction.*** *Substantiate with one or two accomplishments your ability to do the job you are applying for. Build your case in terms as strong as you can make them. Note: The interest and conviction sections, with similar intent, are in some instances interchangeable.*

4) ***Action.*** *A good cover letter needs to move the reader to action. In both sample letters you'll notice that the writer requests an interview. By indicating that you intend to call in person for an interview, you increase your chances of getting it. There's some psychological warfare at work here. A reader who knows a call is coming will feel compelled to deal with the matter in some way, if only to fend off the caller. The point: By making the call you eliminate the possibility of a "passive" rejection. The reader is forced to deal with you, positively or negatively, rather than doom you to a perpetual in-box nondecision.*

Notes on the four elements of an effective cover letter to help you tailor cover letters for specific jobs:

1. **Attention.** Write and refine two or three ways you might capture the reader's attention. *Hint:* One good way is to refer to a prospective employer's need.

    a. ....

    b. ....

    c. ....

2. **Interest.** Write and refine two or three ways to answer the question, "Why should the employer be interested in me?" *Hint:* Emphasize your strong points. Show how your qualities can fulfill the employer's need.

    a. ....

    b. ....

    c. ....

3. **Conviction.** Choose one or two accomplishments that demonstrate the strength of your experience. *Hint:* You'll need to change these for each letter you send, to make them fit the respective situation as closely as possible.

    a. ....

    b. ....

    c. ....

4. **Action.** Write and refine your closing paragraph. *Hint:* Don't leave it up to the prospective employer to call you.

    ....

    ....

    ....

Having done your homework, you are now ready to respond effectively to employment opportunities.

SAMPLE HEALTHCARE RÉSUMÉS AND COVER LETTERS

Résumés and cover letters on the following pages were written by professionals in a variety of healthcare occupations. They have been included to demonstrate:

1) Examples of assertive communication by candidates applying directly to prospective employers
2) Well-worded "Summaries" and "Objectives," and job descriptions that may suggest appropriate phrasing or style for your own résumé
3) Career paths of successful professionals who may have followed somewhat unorthodox job paths to get where they want to go
4) Examples of electronically generated résumés (these are printed in smaller type), included to show you how they appear when printed (and how you might make better use of this medium than others do)

One common characteristic of the healthcare résumés reviewed for this book is a concentration on duties and responsibilities at the expense of accomplishments (as expressed either in the summary or as part of specific job descriptions in the experience section.) Some of these résumés have been printed in their original format, which will enable you to compare them with those résumés that *include* accomplishments. To incorporate the accomplishments that will help you present the most powerful possible image on paper, review page 167 earlier in this chapter. In today's competitive marketplace, including your accomplishments is one way to get the edge over other candidates seeking the job you want.

Sample Cover Letters

The sample letters that follow were generated from a newspaper advertisement and a networking lead, respectively. Examine the two letters point by point for other applications they suggest for your job search.

Newspaper Ad: The classified ads easiest to answer are those that list specific duties as well as position requirements. The more details you have, the easier it will be to demonstrate how closely your background matches the requirements of the job. Notice that the candidate's letter, reprinted on page 174, deals with the position's requirements in the exact sequence they appeared in the ad, reflecting the medical center's presumed priorities.

HEALTHCARE / RADIOLOGY SONOGRAPHER / Full-Time

At Diversey Medical Center, our reputation is based on a commitment to high technology, quality patient care and a strong sense of community. Due to expansion and growth, we are seeking experienced and motivated Sonographers. To qualify, you must be a graduate of an accredited ultrasound program with a minimum of 1 year clinical experience. RDMS registered or registry eligible is required and vascular experience is preferred.

If you're ready to align yourself with a healthcare leader and enjoy a highly competitive compensation and benefits package along with a location easily accessible by public transportation, please send your résumé, including position of interest, to: Laurie Linley, Human Resources, Diversey Medical Center, 7435 W. Damen Ave., Chicago, IL 60631. An Equal Opportunity Employer.

2110 Fabyan Road
Batavia, IL 60131
December 15, 1997

Ms. Laurie Linley
Human Resources Department
Diversey Medical Center
7435 W. Damen Avenue
Chicago, IL 60631
Ref.: Sonographer position

Dear Ms. Linley:

Enclosed is my résumé in response to your December 8 advertisement in the *Chicago Sunday Tribune* for an experienced, motivated sonographer.

First, my experience. I have been employed as staff sonographer at Delnor Hospital since 1989, a position to which I was promoted after serving as a nuclear medicine technologist for two years. I am competent in interpreting anatomic and pathological content, and perform both echocardiographic and general sonographic examinations.

As to my motivation, I am dedicated to a career in medical technology, and have earned four certifications within a four-year period:

* Registered Diagnostic Medical Sonographer - 1987
* Registered Diagnostic Cardiac Sonographer - 1987
* Certified Nuclear Medicine Technologist - 1984
* Registered Technologist (Nuclear Medicine) - 1984

Finally, I know something about Diversey Medical Center's reputation, both from an article in *Chicago* magazine last spring and from an address I heard your administrator, Mr. Kenneth Rivera, make to the Kane County Hospital Association last year.

I look forward to hearing from you and discussing the staff sonographer position at your convenience. I am confident I could make a positive contribution, and help to uphold your justified standing as a leader in the metropolitan Chicago healthcare field.

Sincerely,

Nancy L. Cavallaro

Nancy L. Cavallaro
Enclosure

Networking Lead: Through a former colleague, a recently laid-off medical equipment consultant and former nurse learned of an opening for a cardiology/research nurse at a nearby medical center. After asking questions to learn more about the job and her qualifications for it (her résumé appears on pages 196–197), she called her prospective boss to ask for a personal interview, and followed up with the letter that follows.

---

129 McLeigh Avenue
Englewood, CO 80110
January 14, 1997

Dr. Samuel Insull III
Director of Internal Medicine
Swedish Medical Center
501 E. Hampden Avenue
Englewood, CO 80110

Dear Dr. Insull:

Thank you for your willingness to review my résumé. As I mentioned in our phone conversation, the cardiology/research nurse opening at Swedish Medical Center interests me very much, and is a position I believe I can fill to your satisfaction.

I am an experienced cardiac nurse in both staff and research positions, as you will see from the enclosed résumé. I interact well with doctors, patients, and staff, as my references will attest, and I am comfortable in leadership and administrative roles as well as in a staff position.

My experience at SciMED Life Systems and at the Department of Veterans' Affairs has provided me with excellent experience in the cardiology field—from two quite different perspectives. I played an active role in the cardiac catheterization/angioplasty procedure, and have become very knowledgeable regarding such new technologies as Rotoblator, Excimer Laser, and coronary ultrasound.

Please let me know what additional information I can provide you. In any case I will call next week to see if you agree that a personal interview would be the next best step to determine my qualifications for the cardiology/research position.

Sincerely,

Cassandra Berrian

Cassandra Berrian
Enclosure

PHYSICIANS

Curriculum vitae on the following pages were supplied courtesy of six of the physicians profiled in previous chapters. Many C.V.s include complete lists of publications and presentations, which causes them to run ten pages or longer. For this reason we have printed just one C.V. (radiologist) in its entirety, and edited others down to a length that still illustrates appropriate style and content.

(The two surgeons represented, when asked to cut their C.V.s by 70 percent for space reasons, did so in less than one minute each of "scalpel time"—consistent with job-related decision-making skills they exhibit on a daily basis.)

JANIS M. BROWN

420 Orchard Street
New Haven, CT 06511

203-562-4108 (home)
203-865-1330 (work)

1992 – Present Assistant Professor, Department of Radiology
Yale University School of Medicine, New Haven, CT

Staff Radiologist-Yale New Haven Hospital, New Haven, CT
Veteran's Administration Hospital, West Haven, CT

Certified by the American Board of Radiology

PROFESSIONAL TRAINING:

1991–1992 Yale University School of Medicine/Yale-New Haven Hospital
Cross Sectional Imaging

1988–1991 Yale University School of Medicine/Yale-New Haven Hospital
Resident in General Diagnostic Radiology

1987–1988 Boston University/Mallory Institute of Pathology
Resident in Anatomic Pathology—Autopsy and Surgical
Resident Instructor, Boston University School of Medicine
Department of Pathology

1986–1987 Hartford Hospital, Hartford, CT
Medical/Surgical Internship

EDUCATION:

M.D. Boston University School of Medicine, Boston, MA

M.S. Northeastern University, Boston, MA
Major in Health Sciences

B.S. University of North Carolina, Chapel Hill, NC
Major in Bacteriology

PROFESSIONAL EXPERIENCE:

1980–1982 American Red Cross Blood Services
Coordinator of Special Immune Globulins
Tested, licensed, and marketed hyperimmune globulins including
RhIG and VZIG for passive protection of immunosuppressed patients

1978–1980 Quincy Junior College, Quincy, MA
Instructor in chemistry, biology, and microbiology

Janis M. Brown / 2

AWARDS:

1993   Teacher of the Year—Yale University School of Medicine Department of Radiology

1991   Resident Reporter RSNA/Applied Radiology

1986   Boston University School of Medicine, graduating class of Esther B. Kahn Outstanding Patient Care Award

        Phi Sigma Biology Honor Society

ACADEMIC ACTIVITIES:

Teaching:

Coordinator, Resident Teaching in Ultrasound, Y-NHH

Yale School of Medicine, Medical Student Radiology Course
1989–present

Guest lecturer, Hospital of St. Raphael, New Haven, CT
1992–present

Monthly Conference, Fitkin Medical Service, Y-NHH
1992–present

Annual Radiology Resident Board Review Course,
1993–present

Administrative:

Resident Selection Committee, Y-NHH
1993–present

Space Committee, Y-NHH Radiology
1994–present

Protocol Review Committee, Yale Cancer Center
1995–present

Janis M. Brown / 3

ABSTRACTS:

Hammers LW, Brown J, Scoutt LM, Pellerito JP, Burns G, Taylor KJW: Surveillance with Color Doppler Flow Imaging for Deep Venous Thrombosis in High Risk Trauma Patients. The Radiological Society of North America, 189(P), p226, 1993.

Taylor KJW, Scoutt LM, Quedans-Case C, Pellerito JP, Hammers L, Brown J: Is There a Role for Doppler Imaging in Breast Cancer Diagnosis? The Radiological Society of North America, 169(P) p154, 1993.

Brown JM, Holland CK, Scoutt LM, Taylor KJW: Lower Extremity Volumetric Blood Flow Measurement in Normal Subjects. Journal of US in Med, 14:3 (Suppl) p34, 1995.

Brown JM, Schwartz LB, Taylor KJW, Olive DL: Utero Ovarian Perfusion in Patients Undergoing Ovulation Induction and In Vitro Fertilization. Journal of US in Med, 14:3 (Suppl) p11, 1995.

Lundell A, Taylor KJW, Scoutt L, Brown J, Hammers L, Pellerito J: Optimization of Doppler Parameters in Prediction of Ovarian Malignancy. Journal of US in Med, 14:3 (Suppl) p63, 1995.

Hammers LW, Taylor KJW, Brown JM: Ultrasound Predictors of Spontaneous Resolution in Iatrogenic Peripheral Artery Pseudoaneurysms and Arteriovenous Fistulae. Presented at the American Roentgen Ray Society Annual Meeting, Washington DC, May, 1995 (Session 23, #198).

Brown JM, Taylor KJW, Alderman JL, Quedans-Case C: Contrast Enhanced Visualization of Gonadal Torsion in Dogs using FS-069 Microbubble (MBI). Radiology 197(P), p286, 1995.

Brown JM, Taylor KJW, Alderman JL, Quedans-Case C: Sonographic Visualization of Segmental Organ Perfusion Defects in Dogs using Intravenous Contrast (FS-069). Radiology 197(P), p231, 1995.

Brown JM, Taylor KJW, Alderman JL, Quedans-Case C, Taylor KJW: Enhanced Visualization of Neovascularity in a V×2 Carcinoma by Ultrasonic Contrast (FS069, MBI, Inc.) J Ultrasound Med 15(3) (Suppl) p18, 1996.

Scoutt LM, Taylor KJW, Brown JM, Hammers LW, Restifo RJ: Value of Flow Measurements after Surgical Delay in the TRAM Flaps. J Ultrasound Med 15(3) (Suppl) p9, 1996.

Janis M. Brown / 4

PAPERS:

Brown JM, Hammers LW, Barton J, Scoutt LM, Holland CK, Pellerito J, Taylor KJW. Quantitative Doppler Assessment of Acute Scrotal Inflammation. Radiology, 197:427-431, 1995.

Restifo RJ, Ward B, Scoutt LM, Brown JM, Taylor KJW: Timing, Magnitude, and Utility of Surgical Delay in the TRAM Flap: Part II Clinical Studies. Submitted for Publication, Plastic & Reconstructive Surgery, 1995.

Hammers LW, Cohn S, Brown JM, Burns GA, Scoutt LM, Pellerito JS, Taylor KJW: Doppler Color Flow Imaging Surveillance of Deep Vein Thrombosis in High Risk Trauma Patients. J Ultrasound Med 15:19–24, 1996.

Brown JM, Taylor KJW, Alderman JL, Quedans-Case C, Greener Y: Contrast Enhanced Ultrasound Visualization of Gonadal Torsion. Submitted for Publication, 1996.

Brown JM, Schwartz LB, Olive D, Lange R, Laufer N, Taylor KJW: Evaluation of Doppler Ultrasound as a Means of Monitoring IVF-ET Cycles: Preliminary Results and Findings. Submitted for Publication, 1996.

CHAPTERS AND REVIEWS:

Brown, JM and DiPiro, PJ: High Resolution CT: An Overview. Applied Radiology, Supplement March, 1992; 54–59.

Brown JM, Hammers LW, Rosenfield AR. Scrotal Imaging 1995: Part I, Anatomy and Acute Disease. Applied Radiology, 24(7):27–35, 1995.

Brown JM, Hammers LW, Rosenfield AR. Scrotal Imaging 1995: Part II, Imaging of the Nonacute Scrotum. Applied Radiology, 24(8):23–30, 1995.

Scoutt LM, Brown JM, Hammers LW: Doppler Ultrasound Evaluation of the Native Kidney. Submitted for Publication, Applied Radiology, 1995.

Brown LM, Scoutt LM, Hammers LW: Doppler Ultrasound Evaluation of the Transplant Kidney. Submitted for Publication, Applied Radiology, 1995.

Brown JM, Schwartz LB: Imaging in Ovarian Dysfunction. [IN] Diagnostic Imaging for Reproductive Failure. Parthenon Publishing, NY, In Press.

Dickey KW, Zreik TG, Brown JM, Glickman MG: Imaging and Intervention of the Abnormal Fallopian Tube. [IN] Diagnostic Imaging for Reproductive Failure. Parthenon Publishing, NY, In Press.

Janis M. Brown / 5

INVITED PRESENTATIONS:

Imaging Guided Biopsy of the Abdomen and Pelvis
Clinical Science Lecture Series, Lawrence and Memorial Hospital, New London, CT. January, 1995.

"Ultrasound 1995," Vail, CO. February 1995.
Principles of Hemodynamics—Normal and Disturbed Flow
Color Flow in the Evaluation of Portal Hypertension
Ultrasound Imaging of the Carotid Arteries
Current Status of Breast Imaging

"Doppler Principles and Clinical Applications," Bogota, Colombia. February 1995.
Doppler Evaluation of Portal Hypertension
Imaging of Organ Transplants
Ultrasound Evaluation of the Breast

"Vascular Access—Issues and Interventions," Mystic, CT September, 1995.
Sonographic Evaluation of Dialysis Shunts

"Ultrasound 1996," Breckenridge, CO. February 1996.
Ovarian Masses: Benign and Malignant
Musculoskeletal Ultrasound
Scrotal Ultrasound

RESEARCH IN PROGRESS:

Applications of intravenous contrast in ultrasound studies in animal models.

Measurement of extremity blood flow using Doppler techniques in normal and diseased patients.

Correlation of findings on Captopril scintigraphy, angiography, and renal ultrasound in patients with suspected renal artery stenosis.

Accuracy of imaging studies prior to liver transplant, correlation with explant pathology.

Doppler changes in ectopic pregnancy after treatment with Methotrexate.

CURRICULUM VITAE

DANIEL EDMOND AUSTIN
3015 Pilgrim Lane
Bellingham, Washington 98225
(206) 733-4108 (W); (206) 671-3176 (H)

PRESENT POSITION
Family Physician; North Sound Family Medicine; Bellingham, Washington;
September, 1991 – Present

PROFESSIONAL TRAINING
Family Practice Resident; Providence Family Medical Center; Seattle, Washington;
June, 1988 – June, 1991

EDUCATION
University of California; Santa Barbara, California; B.A. Degree in Mathematics with minor in Physics;
December, 1970
University of Southern California; Los Angeles, California; M.S. Degree in Education; August, 1974
Whitworth College; Spokane, Washington; B.S. Degree in Biology; May, 1984
Dartmouth Medical School; Hanover, New Hampshire; M.D. Degree; June, 1988

CERTIFICATIONS
Diplomate of the National Board of Medical Examiners; July, 1989
Diplomate of the American Board of Family Practice; July, 1991

LICENSURE
Physician & Surgeon License; State of Washington; July, 1990

SOCIETY MEMBERSHIPS
American Academy of Family Physicians
Washington Academy of Family Physicians
Washington State Medical Society
Whatcom County Medical Society
Physicians for Social Responsibility

POSITIONS HELD
Student Representative to Board of Directors of New Hampshire Academy of Family Physicians;
    April, 1985 – June, 1988
Chairperson of Family Medicine Interest Group at Dartmouth Medical School;
    September, 1985 – September, 1986
Member of Committee on Medical Ethics of American Academy of Family Physicians;
    January, 1986 – January, 1987
Member of Committee on Resident and Student Affairs of American Academy of Family Physicians;
    August, 1986 – August, 1988
Alternate Student Delegate of National Conference of Student Members to Congress of Delegates of
    American Academy of Family Physicians; October, 1986
Student Delegate of National Conference of Student Members to Congress of Delegates of American
    Academy of Family Physicians; October, 1986 – September, 1987
Observer to Reference Committee on Public Policy at Congress of Delegates of American Academy of
    Family Physicians; September, 1987

DANIEL E. AUSTIN
page two

POSITIONS HELD (Continued)
Representative to Interorganizational Student Interest Task Force for American Academy of Family Physicians; September, 1987 – October, 1988
Student Observer to Board of Directors of American Academy of Family Physicians; September, 1987 – October, 1988
Chairperson of National Conference of Student Members of American Academy of Family Physicians; September, 1987 – October, 1988
Member of Subcommittee on Resident Working Conditions of American Academy of Family Physicians; January, 1988
Member of Task Force on Student Interest of Board of Directors of American Academy of Family Physicians; April, 1988 – January, 1992
Member of Commission on Legislation and Governmental Affairs of Washington Academy of Family Physicians; January, 1989 – Present
Member of Commission on Legislation and Governmental Affairs of American Academy of Family Physicians; January, 1990 – January, 1992
Member of Pipeline Task Force of Washington Academy of Family Physicians; June, 1991 – Present
Member of Committee on Women in Family Medicine of American Academy of Family Physicians; January, 1992 – January, 1995
Assistant Secretary Treasurer of Washington Academy of Family Physicians; May, 1992 – Present
Co-Chairperson of Commission on Legislation and Governmental Affairs of Washington Academy of Family Physicians; May, 1992 – Present
Member of Committee on Resident and Student Affairs of American Academy of Family Physicians; January, 1995 – Present

PRESENTATIONS
"Medical Ethics Today," Workshop at National Congress of Family Practice Residents and Students of American Academy of Family Physicans; Kansas City, Missouri; August, 1986
"Obstetrics in Family Practice," Workshop at National Congress of Family Practice Residents and Students of American Academy of Family Physicians; Kansas City, Missouri; August, 1989
"An Ounce of Prevention = A Pound of Cure," Workshop at National Congress of Family Practice Residents and Students of American Academy of Family Physicians; Kansas City, Missouri; August, 1990

INTERESTS AND HOBBIES
Family: Spouse, married 22 years; Daughter, age 14; Son, age 11
Fitness Walking
Cross Country Skiing and Hiking
Bicycling
Crossword Puzzles

Curriculum Vitae

NAME: David E. Altobelli

LABORATORY:
Facial Engineering and Morphology Laboratory
Harvard School of Dental Medicine
188 Longwood Avenue
Boston, Massachusetts 02115

EDUCATION:

1978	B.S.	Rensselaer Polytechnic Institute Biomedical Engineering
1982	D.M.D.	Harvard School of Dental Medicine Magna Cum Laude
1985	M.D.	Harvard Medical School

POSTDOCTORAL TRAINING:

Internship and Residencies:

1983–1984	Intern, Oral and Maxillofacial Surgery Massachusetts General Hospital, Boston
1985–1986	Resident, Oral and Maxillofacial Surgery Massachusetts General Hospital, Boston
1986	Resident, General Surgery Massachusetts General Hospital, Boston
1987	Resident, Oral and Maxillofacial Surgery Massachusetts General Hospital The Children's Hospital, Boston, MA
1988	Chief Resident, Oral and Maxillofacial Surgery Massachusetts General Hospital, Boston

LICENSURE AND CERTIFICATION:

1981	National Board of Dental Examinations
1982	Northeast Regional Dental Board
1982	Massachusetts Dental Board Licensure
1987	New Hampshire Dental Board Licensure
1991	Board Certified, American Board of Oral and Maxillofacial Surgery

ACADEMIC APPOINTMENTS:

1991– Present	Director, Facial Engineering Laboratory, Harvard School of Dental Medicine
1991–1994	Assistant Director Research, Division Implant Dentistry Harvard School of Dental Medicine
1988– Present	Instructor in Oral and Maxillofacial Surgery Harvard School of Dental Medicine
1990– Present	Adjunct Professor of Chemical Engineering College of Engineering, Northeastern University
1990– Present	Senior Fellow Center for Biotechnology Engineering, Northeastern University

HOSPITAL APPOINTMENTS:

1988– Present	Associate in Surgery, Brigham and Women's Hospital, Boston
1989– Present	Assistant in Oral Surgery, The Children's Hospital, Boston
1990– Present	Assistant in Oral and Maxillofacial Surgery, Massachusetts General Hospital, Boston
1991– Present	Associate Staff, St. Joseph Hospital, Nashua, NH

AWARDS:

1974	Bausch & Lomb Science Award
1982	Harvard Odontologic Society Award
1982	Student Research Award American Association for Dental Research
1990	National Computer Graphics Association Scholarship
1990, 1991	Nomination for Computerworld Smithsonian Award

MAJOR RESEARCH INTERESTS/PROJECTS:

Three-dimensional imaging/surgical planning—cranio-maxillofacial applications
- Director, Dentofacial Engineering and Morphology Laboratory, HSDM
- Craniofacial Centre clinical team, The Children's Hospital, Boston

In collaboration with SPL, BWH;
- Design and development of three-dimensional computer assisted planning for cranio-maxillofacial surgery
- Craniofacial Morphometric Description
- Intra-operative navigation/enhanced reality for image guided surgery

PUBLICATIONS:
Original Reports

Glowacki, J., Altobelli, D., Mulliken, J., "Fate of mineralized and demineralized osseous implants in cranial defects." Calcif. Tissue Int. 71–76 (1981).

Altobelli, D. E., Lorente, C. A., Handren, J. H., Young, J., Donoff, R. B., and May, J. W. "Free and microvascular bone grafting in the irradiated dog mandible." J.Oral Maxillofac Surg. 45:27–33 (1987)

Altobelli, D. E., Kikinis, R., "Best face forward: New ways to navigate craniofacial surgery." Harvard Medical Alumni Bulletin, Vol. 63 No. 4, (1990)

Motoki, D. S., Altobelli, D. E., Mulliken, J. B., "Enophthalmos following orbital transposition for craniofacial malformations." Plast. Reconstr. Surg. 91:3, 1993

Altobelli, D. E., Kikinis, R., Mulliken, J. B., Cline, H., Lorensen, W., Jolesz, F., "Computer-Assisted Three-Dimensional Planning in Craniofacial Surgery." Plast. Reconstr. Sur. 92:4, 576–585, 1993

Altobelli, D. E. "Computer-Assisted Three-Dimensional Planning for Cranio-Maxillofacial Surgery," Selected Readings in Oral and Maxillofacial Surgery, 3:8, 1–36 (1994) Univ. Texas SW Med. Ctr, Dallas

Movassaghi, K. Altobelli, D. E., Zhou, H., "Frontonasal Suture Expansion in the Rabbit Using Titanium Screws." J. Oral Millofac Surg. 53:1033–1042 1995

Books and Monographs

<u>Encyclopedic Handbook of Biomaterials and Bioengineering</u>, Co-Editors—Wise, D., Trantolo, D., Altobelli, D., Yaszemski, M., Gresser, J., Schwartz, E. Part A: Materials Vols 1,2 pp. 1–1912, Part B: Applications Vols 3,4 pp. 1–1832 Marcel Dekker, Inc., New York, 1995

OBSTETRICIAN/GYNECOLOGIST

Curriculum Vitae

Name: Lowell K. Marbury, M.D.
485 Frontage Avenue
Milford, Connecticut 06460

Military Status: Major, Standby, U.S. Army Reserve (Medical Corps.)
Date of Separation: June 8, 1977

College: New York University, New York, New York
Degree—B.A. (Biology)
Year—1966

Medical School: S.U.N.Y. Downstate Medical Center
Brooklyn, New York
Degree—M.D.
Year—1970

Internship: Bronx Municipal Hospital, Bronx, New York (surgery)
1970–1971

Residency: Mt. Sinai Hospital, New York, New York
1971–1973

The Pennsylvania State University
The Milton S. Hershey Medical Center
Hershey, Pennsylvania
Chief Resident and Clinical Instructor
1973–1975

Board Certification: Diplomate, National Board of Medical Examiners, 1971
Diplomate, American Board of Obstetrics-Gynecology, 1978

Honors Received: Phi Beta Kappa—1966
Honor Scholar, Research in Biochemistry
New York University—1966

Professional Positions: 1979–Present
Private Practice in Obstetrics and Gynecology
Broadside Professional Building
309 Seaside Avenue
Milford, Connecticut 06460
203-877-5634

1979–1983
Consultant Obstetrician-Gynecologist
The Milford Rape Crisis Center
Milford, Connecticut 06460

Lowell K. Marbury, page 2

1978–1979
Director, Obstetrics and Gynecology Services
Department of Obstetrics and Gynecology
Hill Health Center
428 Columbus Avenue
New Haven, Connecticut 06519

1977–1979
Clinical Instructor in Obstetrics and Gynecology
Yale University School of Medicine

1975–1979
Consultant Obstetrician-Gynecologist
Department of Obstetrics and Gynecology
Hill Health Center
428 Columbus Avenue
New Haven, Connecticut 06519

Hospital Appointments: Attending Staff, Yale-New Haven Hospital
Attending Staff, Milford Hospital
Attending Staff, Temple Surgical Center
Courtesy Staff, Hospital of St. Raphael

Societies: Phi Beta Kappa, National Academic Honor Society, 1966
Beta Lambda Sigma, Honor Society in Biology, N.Y.U., 1966
Fellow, American College of Obstetrics-Gynecology, 1979
Member, Connecticut State Medical Society, 1976
Member, New Haven County Medical Society, 1976
Member, Milford Medical Society, 1979
Member, Connecticut Society American Board Obstetricians-Gynecologists, 1979
Member, American Fertility Society, 1980
Member, New England Obstetrical Society, 1981
Member, Society of Gynecologic Laparoscopy, 1993

Licensure: Pennsylvania, New York, and Connecticut

Publications: Extraovular Prostaglandin F a as an Aborticicient in Early Mid-trimester Pregnancy, Robins, J., Marbury, L., et. al. Advances Planned Parenthood Vol. X., No. 1, 1975

Difficult Elective Removal of Majzlin Spring Intrauterine Device. Robins, J., Marbury, L., et. al. Journal of Reproductive Medicine, Vol. 14, No. 2, February, 1975.

Rupture of a Gravid Bicornuate Uterus in a Primagravida Associated with Clostridial and Bacteroides Infection.
Jones, D. E. D., Marbury, L., Journal of Reproductive Medicine, Vol. 21, No. 3, September, 1978

OSTEOPATH

CURRICULUM VITAE

TYLER CHILDS CYMET, D.O.

318 Grower Avenue
Baltimore, Maryland 21209
(410) 627-4113

Personal

Birthdate: January 30, 1963
Birthplace: New York, U.S.A.
Marital Status: Single

Current Position

Ambulatory Medicine—Sinai Hospital of Baltimore
Medical Director—Sinai Community Care
Director of Osteopathic Medical Education

Current Training

Johns Hopkins University/Masters of Science in
Business Program 1996–present

Additional Training

Johns Hopkins Hospital/School of Medicine
Faculty Development Program 1993–1994

Residency

Sinai Hospital of Baltimore 1992–1993
Chief Medical Resident

Yale University School of Medicine 1989–1992
Primary Care Internal Medicine

Internship

Chicago College of Osteopathic Medicine 1988–1989
Rotating Internship/Research Fellowship

Education

Southeastern College of Osteopathic Medicine
Degree Received: D.O. Attended 1984–1988

Northwestern University Medical School 1983

Emory University 1980–1984
Degrees received: B.A. Anthropology,
B.A. Psychology,
Minor in Hebrew Language

Honors

Marquis *Who's Who in America in the South*
Phi Sigma Gamma—Honorary Osteopathic Fraternity
Lambda Alpha—National Anthropology Honor Society
Omicron Delta Kappa—National Leadership Honor Society
Phi Sigma Iota—Foreign Language Honor Society

TYLER CHILDS CYMET, D.O.
page 2

Academic Appointments

    Johns Hopkins University School of Medicine
    Instructor of Medicine 1992–Present

    Kirksville College of Osteopathic Medicine
    Assistant Professor of Internal Medicine
    1994–Present

Grants

    NIH-Primary Care Training Program Grant 1994
    $500,000 yearly x 3 years
    American College of General Practitioners 1988
    $1000
    Merck Sharpe and Dohmo Foundation 1985
    $300
    Dorot Foundation (Research in Political Science) 1981
    $1000

Licensure/Certification

    Florida   1991–Present
    Maryland   1992–Present
    Registered with FDA   DEA
    Advanced Cardiac Life Support Certified (ACLS)
    Advanced Cardiac Life Support Instructor
    Advanced Trauma Life Support Certified (ATLS)
    Pediatric Advanced Life Support Certified (PALS)
    Diplomate: National Board of Osteopathic
        Medical Examiners (NBOME)

Professional Associations

    Maryland Association of Osteopathic Physicians
        1992—CME Coordinator
        1993—Vice President
        1994—President

    American Osteopathic Association
        1992/1993/1994—House of Delegates

    Levindale Hebrew Home for the Aged
        1993–Present—Board of Directors

Experience

    Waterbury Hospital Emergency Room 1990–1992
        Worked part time as an emergency room physician examining and implementing treatment for pediatric, medical and surgical patients in the emergencies department.

    Waterbury Republican-American 1990–1992
        Weekly Columnist, Editorial Writer. Published seventy-two articles on medically related topics.

TYLER CHILDS CYMET, D.O.
page 3

Emory Peer Counseling Center 1980–1984

American Red Cross 1977–1988
  CPR and First Aid Instructor

Skills Fluent in Spanish and Hebrew
Knowledgeable in Computers

Editorial Board

Medical Tribune
1993–present

Hospital Physician
1993–present

Student Doctor
1992–Present, Faculty Advisor
1985–1986 Editor

Urban Medicine
1992–1993

Scientific Articles (Partial list)

"Crohn's disease presenting as massive gastrointestinal bleeding from a gastrocolic fistula," with Paoli Mapelli, M.D. and Eddison Ramsaran, M.D. Journal of the American Osteopathic Association. Accepted 5/92 with revisions, publication pending.

"Ad Diction Ary" of drug users' terms." Journal of the American Osteopathic Association, April 1992, Vol. 92, #4, pages 433–457

"The spread of AIDS in the Haitian-American population: A cultural perspective." Osteopathic Medical News, June 1990, Vol. 7, #6, pages 11–26.

"A lecture on AIDS." Student Doctor, October 1988, Vol. 10, #3, pages 12, 13

"Argyria—Report of a case associated with abnormal electroencephalographic recordings and brain scan findings." Journal of the American Osteopathic Association, July 1987, Vol. 87, #7, pages 509–512. With Mark J. Rosenblatt, D.O.

CURRICULUM VITAE

Stuart Ellis Leland, DVM   Current Address
                            520 Wooster Place
                            New Haven, CT 06511
                            (203) 785-1410

EDUCATION

1984 – 1988	DVM	School of Veterinary Medicine University of California at Davis, Davis, CA Mixed Animal Track
1980 – 1983	BS	College of Agriculture and Life Sciences Cornell University, Ithaca, NY Animal Science with Distinction
1981 – 1982		Biochemistry and Physiology of Farm Animals Reading University, Reading, England Junior Year Abroad

POSTGRADUATE EDUCATION

1994 – present	POSTDOCTORAL FELLOW	Yale University School of Medicine Section of Comparative Medicine New Haven, CT
1988 – 1989	INTERNSHIP	Michigan State University, East Lansing, MI Small Animal Medicine and Surgery Special Interest—Neurology (8-week rotation)

HONORS   1988   The Upjohn Award for Proficiency in Small Animal Veterinary Clinical Medicine

LICENSURE TO PRACTICE

1988 – Present   CALIFORNIA - License number 10871
1990 – Present   WASHINGTON - License number 4155

VETERINARY EXPERIENCE

1993   RESEARCH VETERINARIAN—Regional Primate Research Center University of Washington, Seattle, WA. 50% position providing veterinary and emergency care for 750 – 800 nonhman primates, including neonates and infants, on weekends and holidays.

1991 – 1993   RELIEF VETERINARIAN—Sole proprietor and independent contractor. Managed veterinary practices in Pacific Northwest during owner absence.

1990 – 1991   ASSOCIATE VETERINARIAN—Evergreen Veterinary Hospital, Kirkland, WA. Full-time small animal, four-veterinarian hospital providing emergency service.

Stuart Ellis Leland, DVM / page 2

RESEARCH EXPERIENCE

present   CLINICIAN SCIENTIST—Robert Jacoby, DVM, PhD. Section of Comparative Medicine, Yale School of Medicine, New Haven, CT. Molecular characterization of rat parvoviruses. Development of an *in vivo* model of parvovirus induced oncosuppression.

1993   RESEARCH TECHNICIAN—Chris R. Kaneko, PhD. Department of Physiology and Biophysics, School of Medicine, University of Washington, Seattle, WA. 50% position investigating higher brain control of eye movements in the rhesus monkey.

PROFESSIONAL AFFILIATIONS

American Veterinary Medical Association
Washington State Veterinary Medical Association
American Association for Laboratory Animal Science (AALAS)
Southern New England Branch of AALAS
Scientists Center for Animal Welfare
The American Society of Laboratory Animal Practitioners
Association of Primate Veterinarians

LECTURES/ PRESENTATIONS

1996   *Molecular and In Vivo Studies of a Newly Isolated Rat Parvovirus*
Scientific Platform Presentation National AALAS meeting
Minneapolis, MN

1995   *Biology of Hamsters, Guinea Pigs and Gerbils*
Laboratory Animal Technician Training Course
Yale School of Medicine, New Haven, CT

1994   *Diagnostic Techniques: Serology, Microbiology, Necropsy, Histopathology, Radiology and Radiation*
Southern New England Branch of AALAS
Laboratory Animal Technician Training Course
West Haven, CT

1994   *Anemia and Fever of Unknown Origin in a Juvenile Rhesus (Macaca mulatta).* Association of Primate Veterinarians—Annual Workshop
Pittsburgh, PA

1989   *Thoracic Radiology as a Diagnostic Tool in the Emergency Patient*
Faculty Seminar Series
Michigan State University, East Lansing, MI

PUBLICATIONS

1996   **Leland, S. E.**, Johnson, E. H., Papero, M., Fennie, K. P. A Five Year Retrospective: Bacterial Isolates from Head Cylinder Implants in Macaca spp. *J Med Primatol* (submitted).

1996   Ball-Goodrich, L., Johnson, E. A., **Leland, S. E.**, Nicklas, W., Paturzo, F. X., Smith, A. L., Jacoby, R. O. RPV-1: A Newly Isolated Parvovirus of Laboratory Rats. *J Virol* (submitted).

1996   Johnson, E. H., **Leland, S. E.**, Hotchkiss, C. E. Surgical Correction of an Aberrant Right Subclavian Artery in a Cat. *Contem Top Lab An Sci* (in press).

1994   **Leland, S. E.**, Brownstein, D. G., Weir, E. C. Pancreatitis and Pregnancy Toxemia in a New Zealand White Rabbit. *Contem Top Lab An Sci* 34 (6): 84-5.

NURSES

CASSANDRA BERRIAN
129 McLeigh Avenue
Englewood, Colorado 80110
(303) 468-9954

OBJECTIVE: CARDIOLOGY NURSE—Cardiology research position with direct patient/physician contact

SUMMARY: Experienced cardiac nurse in both staff and research situations. Skilled supervisor, leader, problem solver; ability to interact well with doctors, patients, and staff. Administrative background in budget analysis, scheduling, and admissions. Assertive, creative, and versatile.

EXPERIENCE:

1992 to 1996

SCIMED LIFE SYSTEMS, INC., Maple Grove, MN
<u>Clinical Specialist</u>
- Wrote and presented educational seminars and inservices for physicians, staff, and ancillary personnel in cardiac catheterization/angioplasty laboratory
- Maintained and increased knowledge base on current and new technologies by attending national and regional seminars
- Acted as consultant on product evaluations/introductions, during live-case and other areas of cardiology
- Maintained territory sales level (28% market share) for two five-month periods while sales position was vacant
- Successfully combined products and pricing strategies in response to wide variety of situational client needs

1987 to 1992

VETERANS ADMINISTRATION MEDICAL CENTER, West Haven, CT
<u>Cardiac Clinical Specialist</u> (June 1989 – January 1992)
- Assisted with cardiac catheterization/angioplasty procedure, all setup for procedures, hemodynamic monitoring and medication administration
- Participated in cardiology consult clinic, angioplasty clinic, patient followup and research protocols
- Administered and analyzed budget for cardiac catheterization laboratory; consulted with manufacturers' representatives; scheduled and admitted patients; conducted quality assurance, workload statistics and maintenance of CT surgical cardiac list
- Trained for cross coverage in stress testing, electrophysiology and special procedure radiology
- Compiled and wrote cardiac catheterization manual for JCAHO inspection
- Developed cardiac catheterization/angioplasty teaching program for staff nurses, increasing patient care performance and knowledge base

CASSANDRA BERRIAN
Page 2

<u>Acting Head Nurse</u> (February 1988 – May 1989)
- Organized and maintained daily unit activities; coordinated other services and health care team members
- Supervised staff in clinical decisions; assisted with orientation and preceptorship of new staff
- Improved performance of night nurse through close supervision, reorientation, and developing organizational skills
- Selected as Acting Head Nurse over 15 other nurses

<u>Registered Nurse</u> (April 1987 – January 1988)
- Developed and utilized nursing process for patients in acute medical unit; responsible for physical care, medication distribution, and daily patient activities
- Provided inservices for procedural, equipment, and general disease processes

1986 to 1987

YORK HOSPITAL, York, PA
<u>Graduate Nurse</u>
- Cared for patients with respiratory complications; worked extensively with ventilator dependent patients, tracheotomies, and suction apparatus

EDUCATION: Allentown College of Saint Francis de Sales, Center Valley, PA
<u>B.S. Nursing, 1986</u>

AFFILIATIONS: National League for Nursing

STAFF OR EMERGENCY NURSE (Entry Level)

Don Seigel

1410 Hallowell Drive
Jamestown, North Dakota 58401
(701) 252-7442

OBJECTIVE:

REGISTERED NURSE, Critical Care or Emergency Department Staff

SUMMARY:

* Pediatric Advanced Life Support Provider and Instructor
* Basic Cardiac Life Support Provider and Instructor
* Nationally Registered and North Dakota Licensed EMT-A
* Work effectively with diverse population
* Flexible in meeting patient and unit needs
* Manage time well
* Well-versed in ingestion management, splinting, bandaging, bleeding control, fracture reduction, cervical spine immobilization, and triage

ACCOMPLISHMENTS:

* Presented breakout session on pediatric trauma at American Heart Association conference ("Toward Total Life Support"), Fargo, ND, 1995
* Recipient of state Voiture 40 et 8 nursing scholarship
* Dean's List at University of North Dakota and Fargo Community College
* UND Freshman Academic Scholar
* Historian, Chi Phi Fraternity
* Jamestown Youth Salute Recipient
* Graduated with Honors, Jamestown Senior High School

EXPERIENCE:

CHILDREN'S HEALTHCARE, Fargo, ND   1991 – Present
Emergency Medical Technician, Emergency Department

* Function also as Health Unit Coordinator
* Teach Pediatric Advanced Life Support
* Teach Basic Cardiac Life Support Recertification

UNIVERSITY OF NORTH DAKOTA, Grand Forks, ND   1991
Teaching Assistant, Psychology Department

EDUCATION:

FARGO COMMUNITY COLLEGE, Fargo, ND
Associate Degree, Science in Nursing   1995

UNIVERSITY OF NORTH DAKOTA, Grand Forks, ND
B.A., Psychology (minor in biology)   1991

Sandra L. Nurenburg
114 South Alder Avenue • Elmhurst, Illinois 60147 • (708) 587-6222

SUMMARY

Over 21 years of operating room experience as Manager of Surgery, Charge Nurse, and Staff Nurse. Recognized leader and problem solver who encouraged team building and professional accountability. Outstanding communication and organization skills utilized to maintain effective patient, staff, and physician relationships.

PROFESSIONAL EXPERIENCE

Northwest Memorial Hospital, Chicago, Illinois   1973–1995
A 262-bed hospital

Manager, Surgery (1987–1995)
Responsible for the staffing of 42 employees and coordination of operating room services with 6100 inpatient and outpatient procedures annually. Managed budget of $14 million.
- Created centralized ordering system for department, reducing inventory by 15%–20%.
- Restructured and computerized surgical scheduling and physician preference lists.
- Developed and instituted a peer review program for staff performance evaluations.
- Researched, developed, and staffed an evening shift. (3:00 p.m.–11:30 p.m.)
- Participated in planning for renovation of the operating room, PACU (Post Anesthesia Care Unit), preoperative and postoperative units.
- Partnered with MIS, Patient Accounting and Medical Records to establish a billing system for the Anesthesiologists, resulting in new revenue of $200,000.
- Complied with AORN (Association of Operating Room Nurses) standards and successfully completed two JCAHO (Joint Commission on Accreditation of Healthcare Organizations) reviews.
- Instituted mandatory EKG competency testing for registered nurses, ensuring patient safety.
- Prepared quality improvement quarterly and annual reports.

Charge Nurse, Surgery (1976–1987)
Responsible for daily scheduling, staff assignments, monthly call schedules, purchasing of routine and special equipment, scheduling cases, and evaluation of technical and support staff.

Staff Nurse, Surgery (1973–1976)
Responsible for intraoperative care of the surgical patient.

Oak Park Hospital, Oak Park, Illinois   1972–1973
Staff Nurse, Surgical Unit

Geneva Community Hospital, Geneva, Illinois   1970–1972
Special Procedure Nurse, Radiology (1971–1972)
Charge Nurse, Surgical Unit (1970–1971)

Butterworth Hospital, Grand Rapids, Michigan   1968–1970
Staff Nurse, Medical-Surgical Unit

Sandra L. Nurenburg
Page 2

EDUCATION

BS, Computer Science, 1991
DePaul University, Chicago, Illinois

Nursing Diploma, 1968
Geneva Community Hospital School of Nursing, Geneva, Illinois

PROFESSIONAL AFFILIATIONS

AORN
Illinois Council of Nurse Middle Managers
Geneva Community Hospital School of Nursing Alumni Association

OTHER AFFILIATIONS

Geneva Historical Society Executive Council

Nancy Blumenstein

874 Mill Street
Reno, Nevada 89502

Residence (702) 434-9810
Office (702) 746-4342

Summary

Proven health care professional with over 14 years' experience in progressively responsible health care positions. Known for interpersonal, goal orientation, flexibility, planning, organizational and analytical skills.

Professional History

Reno Children's Hospital, Reno, Nevada   1990–1995

HOME CARE OFFICE RN (temporary), 1994–1995

Performed quality assurance activities to ensure compliance with Joint Commission for Accreditation of Health Care Organizations (JCAHO) regulations.

- Wrote/revised policies and procedures to prepare for accreditation.
- Audited client records to ensure continuing compliance for Quality Assurance.
- Coordinated client services including discharge planning, ordering supplies and client/family teaching.
- Conducted client satisfaction surveys, incorporating results to improve client services when applicable.

STAFFING MANAGER, 1990–1994

Supported quality patient care by continually ensuring adequate staffing levels.

- Eliminated agency usage, saving over $1 million annually by recruiting 60 quality Per Diem Registered Nurses and created support staff pool by crosstraining nurse assistants. This reduced staffing shortages and overtime.
- Implemented computerized scheduling program and automated payroll system for nursing division, saving 5200 man hours annually.
- Formulated steps for computerized interface between payroll and scheduling, which is projected to save $23,000 annually.
- Initiated a Continuous Quality Improvement Process that improved accuracy rate of computerized scheduling by 163% over two years.
- Represented hospital on Flood of 1993 task force.

Foster Quality Care, Reno, Nevada   1988–1990

BRANCH MANAGER

Managed day to day operations of home health and temporary nursing agency, including personnel management, fiscal viability, sales, marketing, program development, policy and procedures, customer relations, quality patient care, and compliance with regulatory agencies.

- Negotiated first ever contracts with five managed care companies, increasing business volume.
- Recipient of divisional award for branch, exceeding bottom line profit for six months.
- Increased agency visits from three to one hundred in one year.
- Turned around collections, reducing accounts receivables from greater than 180 days to less than 90 days.
- Received no deficiencies from surveyors.

Nancy Blumenstein, page 2

Capital Master Home Health Care, Reno, Nevada   1987–1988
ADMINISTRATOR
Started operations for new home health and temporary nursing agency. Recruited all personnel.
- Designed and implemented policies and procedures.
- Created and implemented marketing plan, staying on plan.
- Increased awareness of company by presenting programs to nurses, physicians and community members at large.

DePaul Health Center, Reno, Nevada   1985–1987
ASSISTANT DIRECTOR, STRATEGIC PLANNING   1986–1987
Developed product feasibility studies, physician development plan, Certificates of Need, impact analyses, demographic analyses, competitor profiles, market share analyses, and Strategic Business Plan. Significantly interacted with management, regulatory agencies, and physicians.

ADMINISTRATIVE ASSISTANT to the EXECUTIVE VICE PRESIDENT   1985–1986
Performed special projects including patient complaints, productivity, billing procedures, HMO/PPO proposals, surveys.
- Researched statistical information for all documents, which lead to approval of Certificate of Need, Physician Development Plan, and other decisions made by administration.

Delnor Hospital, St. Charles, Illinois   1980–1984
REGISTERED NURSE   1981–1984
Acute Medicine
Pediatric Intensive Care

ADMINISTRATIVE INTERN (SUMMER)   1980
Conducted special projects in the areas of medical staff credentials, marketing, finance, productivity, ambulatory services, and human resources.

Education
Master of Hospital & Health Care Administration   1983–1985
St. Louis University, St. Louis, Missouri

Bachelor of Science in Nursing   1976–1980
Bradley University, Peoria, Illinois

Professional Memberships
American College of Health Care Executives Diplomate
Reno Women in Health Care Administration

Professional Development
American College of Health Care Executives
Front Line Leadership, Levels I and II
Continuous Quality Improvement, Levels I and II
Social Styles Series

Maria M. Gilmartin
897 Jefferson Boulevard
Santa Fe, New Mexico 87503
(505) 827-1609

SUMMARY:
Twenty years' staff and public health nursing experience. Also offer energy, enthusiasm, self-motivation, teaching skills, demonstrated leadership abilities, and considerable nursing skills.

EMPLOYMENT:

July 1993 to present
Santa Fe Public Health Department
Santa Fe, New Mexico

Public Health Nurse
Responsibilities: Coordinator of NM Bureau of Special Medical Services Child Development Program Clinic. Gather data, make assessment of involved families, arrange appointments, facilitate clinics, assist families to find and secure specialized help for their children, create appropriate reports and do follow-up.

Liaison at Santa Fe Memorial Hospital Birth Place for the "Early Intervention Program" and the Newborn/Post Partum Assessment Home Visit Program.
EIP duties include: Triage post partum discharge summaries to accomplish case finding of high-risk mothers and babies, distribute referrals to appropriate public health nurse and to keep channels of communication open between the hospital and SFPHD.
NB/PP Assessment duties include: Together with the management of the labor and delivery suite of Santa Fe Memorial Hospital set up mechanism to secure referrals for home visits, explain documentation and procedures to the involved public health nurses, distribute referrals to public health nurses and remain available for consult with SFPHD nurses and the hospital staff.

School Nurse—St. Christopher School. Review immunization status of students, carry out vision and hearing screening of students, carry out scoliosis screening as indicated, keep school principal aware of health issues and act as a health consultant for the students, faculty, and the principal.

As a public health nurse I participate in various clinics. For example, Immunization Clinic, HIV/STD Clinics, and seasonal Influenza Clinics.

April 1989 to June 1993
The Haverford Clinic Pediatric Department
Albuquerque, New Mexico

Clinical Supervisor
Accomplishments: Championed a patient-centered focus with support staff. This was accomplished by reorganization, education, and motivation. Authored a course to instruct Certified Medical Assistants in the administration of immunizations currently in use in the Southern Region of The Haverford Clinic. Wrote a Telephone Triage Advice Manual for use in Pediatrics and Family Practice. Participated in the development of The Haverford Clinic Telephone Management Program, an "after hours" triage, advice, and support service.

Maria M. Gilmartin
Page 2

Responsibilities: Day-to-day operation of the Pediatric Department. Orientation of all new employees. All OSHA mandated "Blood-Borne Pathogen" education. Ongoing education and maintenance of OSHA mandated "Exposure Control" plan. Customer relations issues. Interface between Provider staff and Support staff. Educate new parents in "Baby Basics" series of classes.

January 1984 to Present
Cook County Department of Public Health
Skokie, Illinois

Public Health Nurse
As Charge Nurse of the Wheeling Well Baby Clinic, researched and selected a new clinic site, did complete overhaul of clinic schedule and made arrangements for the move. Managed a client caseload in a large geographical area. Did home health care and extensive health teaching. Worked in many clinics, e.g. Employee Health Service, Family Planning Clinic, Prenatal Clinic, Well Child Clinics, Immunization Clinics, and Adult Medical Clinic. Was selected from more than 100 candidates to be one of three nurses in the Cook County Hypertension Screening Team.

October 1982 to December 1983
Vanderbilt University Medical Center
Nashville, Tennessee

Staff Nurse—Neonatal I.C.U.

Head Nurse—Orthopedic Clinic. Promoted to Head Nurse of the Orthopedic Clinic in January of 1983. Did triage and physical assessment, as the clinic served as daytime Ortho Emergency Room. Instrumental in developing the Special Scoliosis Screening Program and clinic.

June 1981 to October 1982
New York University Medical Center
New York City, New York

Staff Nurse—Pediatric I.C.U. General nursing in large teaching hospital Pediatric unit. Promoted twice during tenure. Completed "Team Leadership" training program.

NURSING EDUCATION:
September 1978 to June 1981
Beth Israel Medical Center School of Nursing
* Recipient of the Karpas Award for General Excellence—June 1981

PROFESSIONAL LICENSURE:
Currently hold Registered Professional Nursing licenses in New Mexico, New York, and Illinois

DIETITIAN • OPTOMETRIST • PHARMACIST • SPEECH-LANGUAGE PATHOLOGIST

DIETITIAN

DONNA M. POE, M.S., R.D.
1820 Sixth Street
Wilmington, DE 19805
(302) 871-6322

Educational Background: 1986	**RIH INSTITUTE OF HEALTH PROFESSIONS**, Wilmington, Delaware Master of Science Degree in Dietetics, with concentration in Ambulatory Care Nutrition.
1984 to 1986	**DELAWARE GENERAL HOSPITAL**, Wilmington, Delaware. Dietetic Internship. Rotated throughout hospital, including experience in clinical acute and ambulatory care settings, and food service systems management. Staff relief experience in ICU and step-down units with extensive experience in nutritional assessments, tube-feedings and therapeutic diets.
1986	**HARVARD UNIVERSITY EXTENSION**, Cambridge, Massachusetts. Marketing and business writing courses in fulfillment of master's degree.
1980	**UNIVERSITY OF VERMONT**, Burlington, Vermont. Bachelor of Science Degree, Major: Dietetics with professional emphasis in Nutrition Education.
Professional Development: 1990 to present	**NUTRITION CONSULTANT:** Self-employed. Provide a variety of nutrition-related services including personalized nutrition counseling in a private-practice setting, with special interest in sports nutrition and weight management. Developed and presented successful weight management program at Hampshire Hills Sports & Fitness Club, Wilmington, Delaware. Conduct corporate and community seminars, lead supermarket tours, consult to home health care agency, and perform computerized recipe analysis for small business.
1986 to 1990	**OUTPATIENT CLINICAL DIETITIAN:** Emerson Hospital, Wilmington, Delaware. Counseled clients on normal and therapeutic diets utilizing self-designed patient education materials, and lectured in corporate and community settings. Developed in-patient and out-patient coronary teaching classes on nutrition and heart disease, and created successful 10-week "Stressless Weight Loss Program," including body composition analysis using bioimpedence analyzer. Full-time.
1986 (Jan.-Sept.) part-time	**PROGRAM ASSISTANT: EATING FOR THE HEALTH OF IT**, Delaware General Hospital, Wilmington, Delaware. Researched and developed student manual for 8-week health promotion program and analyzed nutrient intake of clients on IBM-PC.
1986 (Apr.-Aug.) part-time	**DIETITIAN:** Elliot Hospital, Wilmington, Delaware. Assessed nutrient needs and counseled patients, with primary responsibility in cardiac and radiation therapy units. Developed instructional materials for in-patient and out-patient use.
1986 (Jan.-May) part-time	**NUTRITION EDUCATOR:** Wilmington-Cambridge Elder Services, Wilmington, Delaware. Coordinated elderly recipe contest/fitness festival based on U.S. Dietary Guidelines, which was attended by 800+ elders. Responsible for recruitment of judges, volunteers, contestants and exhibitors. Developed participative game show to promote good nutrition, which was filmed for local cable TV show.

Donna Poe, page 2

1985 (temporary)	**CLINICAL DIETITIAN:** Massachusetts General Hospital, Boston, Massachusetts. Assessed nutritional needs of patients, developed and implemented nutrition care plans, counseled patients, and supervised nutrition assistants. Primary responsibility in ICU and Orthopedic units.
1981 to 1984	**DIETETIC TECHNICIAN:** Donald N. Sharp Memorial Hospital, San Diego, California. Assisted patients in menu selection, counseled patients and families, participated in team rounds and conferences in the Rehabilitation Center, and supervised food service personnel. Coordinated nutrition component of cardiac rehabilitation program with chief clinical dietitian, including development of slides and hand-out materials.
1980	**NUTRITION EDUCATION INTERNSHIP:** H.O. Wheeler Elementary School, Newark, Delaware. Planned, taught and promoted nutrition for Project Follow Through, a federally-funded program. Produced a collection of nutrition education materials for teachers, parents and children.
Professional Organizations:	Member of the American Dietetic Association. Dietetic Practice Groups: Sports Cardiovascular & Wellness Nutritionists and Nutrition Entrepreneurs Member of the Delaware Dietetic Association, Board of Directors DDA Profile Editor, 1993—present Member of the Professional Education Committee of the American Cancer Society, Delaware Division, Walden Unit, 1986–1990
Publications & Media:	"Food Habits and Nutritional Knowledge of Portuguese Participants in an Elderly Nutrition Program." Journal of Nutrition for the Elderly, Vol 12: 1, 1992. "Creating Quality Presentation Materials On A Shoestring Budget"; Presentation at New Hampshire Dietetic Association, Fall Meeting, 1991. *Profile of Portuguese Elderly Nutrition Program Participants: Demographic Characteristics, Nutrition Knowledge, and Practices.* University Microfilm International: Ann Arbor, Michigan, 1988. "Gameshow Promotes Nutrition Education for Elders." Journal of Nutrition Education, 19: Gem No. 82, 1987. "Demographic Characteristics and Nutrition Knowledge of Portuguese Elders Participating in an Ethnic Nutrition Program." The American Dietetic Association, 69th Annual Meeting, Las Vegas, Nevada. Poster Session and Abstract. October, 1986. Newspaper articles and radio talk show guest on a variety of nutrition topics for local papers/radio station.
References:	Furnished upon request.

OPTOMETRIST

STEPHEN J. HARNEY, O.D., F.A.A.O.
3953 Bartlett Street
Providence, Rhode Island 02860

EDUCATION
1978   Doctor of Optometry
        New England College of Optometry, Boston, Massachusetts
        (Presently fulfilling requirements for T.P.A. Certification)
        Rhode Island License #945, T.P.A. Certified

1974   Bachelor of Arts in Biology
        Saint Anselm College, Manchester, New Hampshire

EMPLOYMENT EXPERIENCE

BARTLETT EYE CLINIC, INC., Providence, Rhode Island
A large multi-satellite ophthalmology practice, which offers comprehensive eye care services.

July 1978 to Present

Director, Contact Lens Clinic
Full responsibility for all aspects of contact lens services. Clinical responsibilities include the evaluation, fitting and follow-up of contact lens patients. Expertise in fitting daily wear and extended wear soft lenses (aphakic and cosmetic), gas permeable lenses and specialty lenses (torics, bifocal contacts, etc.). Particular interest and competence in fitting the most difficult cases (keratoconus, disfigured pupils, etc.). Periodic involvement in investigational contact lens research.

Administrative responsibilities include the purchasing of all contact lens related materials and involvement in the hiring and supervising of staff optometrists and ophthalmic technicians.

July 1978 to Present

Director, General Optometry Department
Perform general optometric services including pediatric and geriatric care with emphasis on pathological diagnosis and management; clinical advisor to staff optometrists.

July 1978 to Present

Director, Ultrasound Department
Perform various diagnostic and follow-up procedures by A-scan ultrasound. Particular emphasis on axial length determination for lens implants.

September 1989 to Present

Adjunct Clinical Instructor, New England College of Optometry in cooperation with Bartlett Eye Clinic, Inc.
Instruct and advise senior optometric interns in all phases of contact lens and optometric clinical care at Bartlett Eye Clinic, Inc.

NORTH SHORE EYE SPECIALISTS, Danvers, Massachusetts
A highly skilled general optometric practice with special interests in the field of contact lenses, low vision, and pediatrics.

HARNEY/ 2

February 1991 to April 1995
Associate and Contact Lens Specialist
Utilized years of contact lens and medically related experience to evaluate and manage an array of ocular conditions with special emphasis on contact lens related cases.

RHODE ISLAND EYE INSTITUTE OF THE RHODE ISLAND COLLEGE OF OPTOMETRY, Providence, Rhode Island
A teaching affiliate of the Rhode Island College of Optometry

March 1995 to Present
Adjunct Assistant Clinical Professor
Instruct and advise junior and senior optometric interns in all phases of clinical contact lens care.

LEXINGTON EYE ASSOCIATES, Newport, Rhode Island
A large multi-satellite ophthalmology practice, which offers comprehensive eye care services.

April 1995 to September 1995
Consultant, Contact Lens Clinic
Interim consultant and contact lens clinician using years of medically related contact lens experience to evaluate, manage and advise on an array of challenging and complicated contact lens conditions concentrating in the area of rigid gas permeable and specialty designs (torics, bifocal contacts, etc.)

Consulting responsibilities also included advice regarding contact lens management and administrative decision making.

MICROSURGICAL EYE CONSULTANTS, Providence, Rhode Island
An ophthalmology practice, which offers comprehensive eye care services.

December 1995 to Present
Director, Contact Lens and Optometric Services
Full responsibility for the development and management of a newly formed contact lens and optometric service. The responsibilities include clinical, administrative, and advisory capacities.

CONTINUING EDUCATION
Annual attendance at American Academy of Optometry Convention
Annual attendance at Rhode Island Council of Optometry Convention
Attendance at selected seminars offered by the Rhode Island Society of Optometrists and the Rhode Island College of Optometry

PROFESSIONAL
Candidate: Cornea and Contact Lens Diplomate - A.A.O.
Fellow: American Academy of Optometry
Member: Rhode Island Chapter - A.A.O.
Member: American Optometric Association
Member: Contact Lens Section - A.O.A.
Member: Rhode Island Society of Optometrists

REFERENCES Available upon request

GEORGE BOWERSOX
461 Allen Avenue
Nashua, New Hampshire 03051
(603) 471-6080

SUMMARY

- More than fifteen years of Pharmacy experience in retail and hospital settings.
- Technical knowledge and capability is enhanced by strong communication skills which facilitate the development of positive relationships with customers and medical professionals.

EXPERIENCE

1978–Present *WHITNEY PRESCRIPTION PHARMACY, Nashua, NH*
Director of Pharmacy Operations & Pharmacist-In-Charge
- Prepare and dispense medications prescribed by physicians, dentists, and veterinarians including compounded medications not commercially available.
- Provide information and counsel to customers and medical professionals.
- Recruit, select, train, supervise, schedule, and evaluate Staff Pharmacists for three retail locations.
- Utilize, maintain, and upgrade computer hardware and software including customized and widely used applications such as Microsoft Windows and Excel.
- Co-authored company Policies and Procedures manual.
- Set up, competitively priced, and managed drug formulary of over 3000 drug products.

1987–1992 (part-time) *BROOKSIDE HOSPITAL, Nashua, NH*
Staff Pharmacist
- Five years' hospital experience including unit dose dispensing, inventory control, drug information retrieval, and nursing station inspection.

1971–1978 *WORLD'S FAIR PHARMACY, Flushing, NY*
Pharmacy Intern

EDUCATION

B.S., Pharmacy, BROOKLYN COLLEGE OF PHARMACY, 1978
A.A., CITY UNIVERSITY OF NEW YORK at Queens, 1975

AFFILIATIONS

Chairman, Nashua Pharmacists Assembly
Member, National Association of Retail Druggists

JANET B. DAVIS
1401 Kaneville Road
Amherst, Massachusetts 01237

OBJECTIVE
Seeking a challenging position in the field of rehabilitation/healthcare.

July 1992 – Present: Open Horizon Children's Centers, Amherst, MA
Speech/Language Pathologist
Responsible for providing direct evaluation and treatment to pre-school and elementary children on a one-to-one basis and in integrated classroom settings. Also carried an early intervention (birth to three years) caseload. Population comprised of Down Syndrome, Cerebral Palsy, PDD, and ADD individuals; multiple handicapped, and speech/language delayed. Other responsibilities: Community inservice education, health/wellness screenings, "guest" speaker appointments at local elementary, middle, high schools, and junior college.

Souhegan High School, Amherst, MA
Speech/Language Pathologist-contract
Responsible for providing direct service (treatment and evaluation) to senior high school students, as well as consultation to classroom teachers and advisors.

April 1990 – July 1992: St. Michael's Hospital/New England Rehabilitation Center, Greenfield, MA
Referral Specialist
Coordinated admissions to the rehabilitation center in Springfield, MA, and to a sub-acute center in Boston, MA. Responsibilities included: pre-admission screening evaluation; sales and marketing of product lines, patient/family education; physician, and insurance case manager contact. Responsible for coordinating regional educational inservice offerings and assisting with new program development.

March 1988 – March 1990: Tri-City Medical Center, Oceanside, CA
Rehabilitation Admissions Liaison
Responsible for coordinating admissions to the rehab unit. Specific Responsibilities: pre-admission screening; family education; physician, insurance case manager and discharge coordinator contacts. Also, utilization review, quality assurance, and program development.

Meridian NeuroCare, Escondido, CA
Speech/Language Pathologist
Provided speech/language services to primarily head-injured population, in a small, private, skilled nursing facility. Contractual basis. Evaluation and treatment of speech, language, voice, and swallowing disorders. Provided staff inservices.

_____ Janet B. Davis/2 _____

May 1986 – March 1988: Shea Products, Inc., Rochester, MI
Account Representative
Participated in development of advertising/marketing for Shea Products' "Special Friend" communication device for non-oral children and adults. Responsible for marketing and sales in California and Australia.

EDUCATION
M.S., University of Michigan, Speech/Language Pathology, 1985
B.S., University of Michigan, Speech/Language Pathology with Psychology/Spanish minor, 1984

CERTIFICATIONS/LICENSURE
1994   Massachusetts State Licensure
1986   California State Licensure
1986   California Provisional Teaching Certification
1985   Michigan Provisional Teaching Certification

PROFESSIONAL AFFILIATIONS
American Speech/Language and Hearing Association
Kappa Delta Pi Educational Honor Society

ALLIED HEALTH PROFESSIONALS

MICHAEL LAYTON
1671 Alabaster Highway • Uvalde, Texas 78801
(512) 276-5186

OBJECTIVE: CARDIAC CATHETER LAB MANAGEMENT

SUMMARY: Experienced in invasive/non-invasive cardiology, cardiac catheterization/pacemaker implantation, electrophysiology studies, exercise stress testing, Holter scanning, EKG, pacemaker follow-up, cardiac rehabilitation/prevention, staff training and supervision, clinical trials, computer interface, input, output and analysis, yearly budgets, capital acquisitions, vendor negotiations.

EQUIPMENT USED: Honeywell Meddars 300; PPG 1280; Datascope Intra Aortic Balloon Pump; Hewlett Packard Arrhythmia Monitoring System; Cinerex Film Processor; Vanguard Projector; Medtronic, Telectronics Pacemakers; Quinton 5000 Scanner

EXPERIENCE:

1992 TO PRESENT   HAPPY VALLEY PHYSICIANS' HOSPITAL, Austin, TX
Cardiology Supervisor
- Hire and train staff
- Provide educational support to cardiac services and ancillary departments
- Write and maintain policies, protocols and standards, quality improvement, and budgets
- Supervise invasive and non-invasive cardiology procedures
- Maintain federally mandated implantable medical device reports

1987 TO 1992   COMMUNITY HOSPITAL, Austin, TX
Invasive Cardiology Registered Nurse (1989–1992)
- Performed and assisted in non-invasive and invasive procedures
- Managed in/outpatient pacemaker/AICD clinic under indirect guidance of physician; started and maintained implantable defibrillator support group
- Performed data collection and analysis necessary for clinical care areas
- Assisted in bringing new non-invasive and invasive procedures to department

Staff Registered Nurse—Coronary/Intensive Care Unit (1987–1989)
- Provided primary nursing care with use of invasive hemodynamic monitoring
- Provided on-call nursing care for acutely ill patients undergoing invasive cardiology procedures
- Oriented and trained newly hired personnel

EDUCATION: SYRACUSE UNIVERSITY, Syracuse, NY
1985—B.S., School of Nursing

CERTIFIED REGISTERED NURSE ANESTHETIST

James Lee Hawes, CRNA
22645 County Road 440
Oakland, Iowa 51560

SUMMARY:	Experienced with general, orthopedic, pediatric, obstetric, neurovascular, thoracic, and emergency ASA I-IV patients. Responsible for administering intravenous, inhalation, regional (SAB and Bier Blocks), and MAC anesthesia. Able to work with or without M.D. anesthesiologist. Provide both pre-and post-anesthesia assessment.
EXPERIENCE:	
1992 to Present	MEDICAL ANESTHESIA ASSOCIATES, Council Bluffs, IA
Staff CRNA
–Provide anesthesia services for Jennie Edmundson Hospital
1988 to 1992	SHELBY BOUNTY MYRTLE MEMORIAL HOSPITAL, Harlan, IA
Anesthetist
–Provided anesthesia services for small rural hospital
1987	McDOWELL HOSPITAL, Marion, NC
Freelance Anesthetist
–Provided anesthesia coverage and help for small community hospital
1974 to 1987	WESTERN NC ANESTHESIA ASSOCIATES, Asheville, NC
Staff CRNA
–Provided anesthesia services for St. Joseph's Hospital (300 beds)
1973 to 1974	NORTH MEMORIAL HOSPITAL, Minneapolis, MN
Anesthetist
–Provided services for large city hospital. Also freelance anesthetist at Golden Valley (MN) Hospital
1969 to 1971	U.S. NAVY NURSE CORPS
Charge Nurse, Pediatrics, Orthopedics, and Psychiatry
–Supervisor, Pediatric out-patient department
1969	NEBRASKA METHODIST HOSPITAL, Omaha, NE
Staff Nurse, Intensive Care Unit
EDUCATION:	UNIVERSITY OF IOWA, Iowa City, IA
Pursuing external Bachelor's Degree, majoring in sciences

CREIGHTON UNIVERSITY, Omaha, NE
1995—Trauma Seminar and Hands-On Central Line Workshop

DANNEMILLER MEMORIAL EDUCATION ASSOCIATION, San Antonio, TX
1984—Nurse Anesthetist Review Course and Hands-On Spinal Workshop

MINNEAPOLIS SCHOOL OF ANESTHESIA, Minneapolis, MN
1973—Diploma in Nurse Anesthesiology

NEBRASKA METHODIST SCHOOL OF NURSING, Omaha, NE
1969—Diploma in Professional Nursing

Continuing Education Programs: AANA Journal Continuing Education Course; current reviews for Nurse Anesthetists; on-going CEU course and various drug company CEU courses |
| **PROFESSIONAL ASSOCIATIONS:** | American Association of Nurse Anesthetists
RN License in Iowa, Minnesota, and North Carolina
Advanced Registered Nurse Practitioner in Iowa |

DIRECTOR OF RADIOLOGY

ROBERT S. TINNON
14041 Sepulveda Boulevard
Los Angeles, California
(213) 888-2212

OBJECTIVE: Radiology Department Director

SUMMARY: Twenty-two year background in imaging, including fourteen years radiology department supervision. Extensive responsibility for capital and operating budgets, personnel management, equipment selection, and compliance with government agency standards.

EXPERIENCE:

1992 to Present
RIVERSIDE COMMUNITY HOSPITAL, Riverside, CA
Radiology Supervisor
* Supervise staff of 11 in 360-bed acute care facility
* Completed capital and operating budgets for 1996
* Manage departments of diagnostic x-ray, ultrasound, nuclear medicine, CT, radiation oncology, and radiologic technology school

1988 to 1992
WASHINGTON MEDICAL CENTER, Culver City, CA
Interim Director, Radiology
* Marketed imaging services to local physicians
* Coordinated ACR accreditation of mammography facility
* Participated in Customer Service Committee
    —improved overall department rating to 97% favorable
* Consistently successful in JCAHO surveys

1985 to 1988
COMMUNITY MEMORIAL HOSPITAL, Menominee Falls, WI
Chief Technologist, Radiology
* Performed administrative and department director functions
* Supervised staff of six technologists in CT, cardiac cath, angiography, and ultrasound

1983 to 1985
GUNDERSEN CLINIC, Two Rivers, WI
Staff Radiologic Technologist

EDUCATION: UNIVERSITY OF WISCONSIN, Madison, WI
1981—B.S., Health Sciences
1983—Certificate, Lutheran Hospital School of Technology

PROFESSIONAL AFFILIATIONS: American Healthcare Radiology Administrators
American Registry of Radiologic Technologists
American Society of Radiologic Technologists
Radiology Administrators of SE Wisconsin, President, 1988

LABORATORY TECHNICIAN (Entry Level)

KARI LYNN WILSON
155 Graham Street • Stratford, Tennessee 37716 • (615) 381-9443

OBJECTIVE:

BIOTECHNOLOGY LABORATORY POSITION
WITH OPPORTUNITY FOR GROWTH

SUMMARY:

Recent graduate (B.S. Biology/Chemistry) with good computer, interpersonal, and communication skills. Strong work ethic, reliable, detail-oriented. Excellent lab skills. Work well both independently or in team situations.

LABORATORY SKILLS:

Pour plating; spread plating; petrifilm; api strip; incubation plates; stomacher; dilution schemes; tube inoculation; pipeting; gram staining; anerobe jar; spectrometer

EDUCATION:

University of Tennessee, Knoxville, TN
1996 - B.S., Biology major; Chemistry minor
    3.1 GPA in major
    Intramural sports; U of Tenn Fitness Club
    * Paid for 80% of school costs through summer and meal jobs

EXPERIENCE:

Summer, 1994 - Volt Temporary Services, Memphis, TN
    Assigned to work in food distribution center for area wholesalers: Learned to interact successfully with wide variety of individuals.

Summer, 1993 - Diversey Engineering - Assisted in sanitizing equipment utilized in pasteurization processes: Worked effectively as part of team.

Summer, 1992 - Lewis Construction Company - Assisted new contractor keeping time sheets and scheduling projects. Suggested several new procedures that were adopted by employer.

PHYSICAL THERAPIST

SALLY J. SPATAFORA
710 Grove Beach Road North
Westbrook, Connecticut 06498
203-681-4120

OBJECTIVE   PHYSICAL THERAPY MANAGEMENT

SUMMARY
Thirteen years' physical therapy experience, including five years of management and supervisory responsibilities. Skilled in administering outpatient orthopedics involving work-related and athletic injuries, post-surgical rehabilitation, neck, and back care. Background in community outreach programs for students interested in physical therapy as a career.

WORK EXPERIENCE
February 1991–January 1996
Assistant Supervisor, Temple Physical Therapy, New Haven, CT.
Responsibilities included:
- 60% patient care of outpatient orthopedics involving: work-related injuries, athletic injuries, post-surgical rehabilitation, neck and back care
- Center Clinical Coordinator, five years
- Scheduling of 10–20 physical therapists
- Presentation of a monthly Back School class in the clinic and community
- Clinical supervision of all staff physical therapists
- Physical therapist in Work Conditioning Program
- Coordination of an observation program involving area high school students and individuals interested in pursuing a career in physical therapy
- Head Committee on peer and utilization reviews
- Assistance in daily operations of Temple Physical Therapy involving 60 employees, 2 offices, and several related programs including aquatic rehabilitation, work hardening, cardiac rehabilitation, and exercise.

June 1995–August 1995
Academic Coordinator of Clinical Education, University of Connecticut, Storrs, CT. Part time, acting ACCE responsible for physical therapy students on clinical affiliation.

May 1987–February 1991
Assistant Supervisor, Temple Physical Therapy, Hamden, CT.
Responsibilities included:
- 70% patient care
- Scheduling of approximately seven physical therapists
- Presentation of monthly Back School classes in the clinic and community
- Recruiting and scheduling weekly inservices
- Coordination of observation program
- Assist in daily operation of Temple Physical Therapy satellite office
- Responsibility of all operation in the supervisor's absence

August 1983–May 1987
Staff Physical Therapist, Temple Physical Therapy, New Haven and Hamden, CT.
Primary responsibilities included patient care with experience in athletic screening, clinical instructor and development of the Back School program.

SALLY J. SPATAFORA
PAGE 2

EDUCATION
1983	B.S., Physical Therapy, University of Connecticut, Storrs, CT
1977–1979	Classes in Allied Health and Environmental Studies, Johnson St. College, Johnson, VT

CONTINUING EDUCATION
- 1984 — Advance Manual Orthopedics, Cyriax, Quinnipiac College, 3 cr., Ross Woodman, PT
- 1984 — T.E.N.S., CAPTA
- 1984 — Isokinetic workshop, Cybex
- 1985 — Introduction to Evaluation and Mobilization of the Spine, Institute of Graduate Health Science
- 1985 — Work Capacity Evaluation
- 1986 — Diagnosis and Treatment of the Trunk and Extremities—Indirect Techniques, Loren H. Rex, DO, USRA Foundation
- 1986 — Clinical Electrotherapy, CAPTA, Joseph Kahn, PhD
- 1987 — Advanced Evaluation and Mobilization of the Cranio-facial, Cervical, and Upper Thoracic, Institute of Graduate Health Science
- 1987 — Introduction to Muscle Techniques, Loren H. Rex, DO, USRA Foundation
- 1987 — Diagnosis and Treatment of Muscle Imbalances Associated with Musculoskeletal Pain, Shirley Sahrmann, PhD
- 1987 — The Pelvis: Function and Dysfunction Treatment with Muscle Energy Techniques and Indirect Techniques, CAPTA, Sharon Weiselfish, PT
- 1988 — Myofacial Release, Robert Ward, DO
- 1988 — Introduction to Craniosacral Therapy, Upledger Institute
- 1989 — Intermediate Craniosacral Therapy, Upledger Institute
- 1989 — Emerging Theories of Liability in the Workplace, AAIM
- 1989 — Interpersonal Effectiveness, Center for Creative Change, evenings 12 hours
- 1989 — How to Supervise People, Fred Pryor
- 1989 — Applying Acupuncture Principle to Bodywork, Upledger Institute
- 1989 — Manual Medicine of the Cervical and Thoracic Spine, Ed Stiles, DO
- 1990 — The Shoulder in Sports, Annual Yale Sports Medicine Seminar
- 1990 — Quality Assurance Workshop, APTA
- 1991 — The Role of the Clinician as Clinical Educator, New England Consortium of ACCE
- 1991 — Anatomic Basis for Differential Diagnosis of Somatic Dysfunction, Carl Steele, PT, DO
- 1992 — Musculoskeletal Evaluation and Treatment: Standardization of Essential Muscle Length and Strength Tests, Florence P. Kendall, PT
- 1992 — Human Anatomy Review Course, Upper Extremity and Cervical Region, CPTA
- 1993 — Evaluation and Management of the Temporomandibular Disorders, Steven Kraus, PT, OCS
- 1993 — Evaluation and Management of Cervical Dysfunction, Steven Kraus, PT, OCS
- 1993 — Musculoskeletal and Sports Rehabilitation Focus: Disorders of the Rotator Cuff, The Physical Medicine and Rehabilitation Center, PA
- 1993 — Rehabilitation Psychology and Pain Management, Mitchell J. Cohen, MD and Robert D. Thrift, EdD

PROFESSIONAL ORGANIZATION
American Physical Therapy Association, Orthopedic Chapter

X-RAY TECHNICIAN

Samuel D. Smith
912 S. Snodgrass Street
Portland, Oregon 97209
(503) 221-0604

SUMMARY

Nine years' experience in fluoroscopic, orthopedic and standard x-ray procedures—in military and civilian hospitals. Background in both orthopedic and urgent care facilities. Wide range of back-office skills, including the application of fiberglass casting.

WORK HISTORY

Drs. Harris/Bliss/Kay and Hollander
Portland, OR
(503) 486-1686
March 1995–Present
Orthopedic back office

Orthopedic Medical Center
Oregon City, OR
(503) 481-0168
January 1994–March 1995
X-ray Tech/Orthopedic Tech

First Care Medical Group
Lake Oswego, OR
(503) 444-2168
February 1993–January 1994
X-ray Tech/Medical Assistant

Orthopedic Services Dr. Robert Cratchett
410 Winery Ave.
Ashland, OR
November 1991–January 1994
X-ray Tech

Henry Mayo Newhall Hospital
23845 W. McBean Parkway
Valencia, CA 91355
July 1988–October 1992
X-ray/Fluoroscopy Tech

EDUCATION

BA – The Master's College
CRT RHT 91431 – USAF School of Health Care Sciences
ARRT – (exam eligible/test date March 1998)

REFERENCES

Available on request.

HEALTHCARE EXECUTIVES

CLAY JORDAN
410 Nighttrain Lane
Escanaba, Michigan 49807

Office: (906) 324-3112　　　　　　　　　　　　　　　　Fax: (906) 324-2101

SUMMARY

Sixteen years' experience in marketing, US and international sales, strategic planning and business development with five major *in vitro* diagnostics companies; a strong technical background; proven ability to lead existing or form new groups during periods of change.

PROFESSIONAL EXPERIENCE

MILLER DIAGNOSTICS INC. (Technicon Instruments Corp.)　　1992–Present
$1 billion diagnostic company following the merger of Miles and Technicon in mid-1993.

Vice President, Planning and Business Development (1994–Present)
- Prepared strategic plan for $300 million chemistry and immunochemistry businesses.
- Managed major alliance with Toshiba Corporation and used negotiating ability to convert it from a confrontational to a more cooperative relationship.

Vice President, Marketing (Technicon, North American Division) (1992–1994)
$200 million Division prior to acquisition
- Managed Marketing, Telemarketing, Creative and Technical Groups with 50 people and $8 million advertising and promotion budget.
- Reorganized and refocused Marketing Department, achieving strong market segment orientation.
- Revitalized advertising approaches, including selecting new advertising agency resulting in improved customer perception.
- Controlled spending on advertising, saving $750 thousand without losing customer impact.
- Directed the launch of six major products, replacing and expanding entire product line.
- Active member of integration team following merger that designed and proposed marketing and sales organizations.

CLAY JORDAN
Page 2

PENTAX CLINICAL INSTRUMENTS   1989–1992
New division of Pentax Corporation formed to market Japan-manufactured clinical analyzers directly to US hospitals and clinical laboratories.

Director of Marketing
- One of team of three who planned and established new division, which achieved first year sales of $33 million.
- Proposed structure and implemented the prioritized and staged growth of organization that grew to over 100 people within 2 years.
- Successfully negotiated early termination of distribution agreement, OEM contract and University affiliation, with immediate $6 million revenue and long term product flow.
- Achieved 100% market share in chain commercial laboratories and over 50% share in large blood collection centers by sharp targeting and positioning.
- Created a separate business to market the biotechnology products of a joint venture company.

GIFFORD INSTRUMENTS CORPORATION (Corning)   1986–1989
$40 million company acquired by Corning in 1983.

Director, International Sales and Marketing (1987–1989)
- Introduced and drove the sale of Gifford products through the international Corning Medical organization following the acquisition.
- Developed plans and implemented the introduction of five new products simultaneously worldwide.
- Consistently met $12 million sales budget during period of overall declining sales.

Director, Market Development (1986–1987)
- Formulated strategic plans that positioned company for future growth.
- Focused product development resulting in the EXPRESS, a product that achieved 30% market share and sales of over $20 million.

CLAY JORDAN
Page 3

BOEHRINGER MANNHEIM DIAGNOSTICS (Houston, Texas)   1983–1986
$35 million Hycel company acquired in 1979 and merged with Boehringer Mannheim Corporation.

Product and Group Product Manager (1984–1986)
- Marketed the large clinical chemistry systems which justified the acquisition.

Manager, Instruments Evaluations (1983–1984)
- Applied the Boehringer Mannheim reagents to the Hycel instruments in less than six months.

BECKMAN INSTRUMENTS (Houston, Texas)   1980–1983
$400 million diagnostics and analytical systems company.

Medical Systems Specialist
- As part of field sales organization, provided technical support to sales force and customers.
- Grew RIA business from $200 thousand to $2.5 million in 2.5 years.

EDUCATION

Post Doctoral Fellow, Tulane College of Medicine, Houston, Texas - 1980
Ph.D. in Biochemistry, University of Tennessee - 1977
AB in Chemistry, Asbury College, Wilmore, Kentucky - 1971

HOSPITAL ADMINISTRATOR

THELMA L. CUMMINGS

175 West 73rd Street, #8G
New York, NY 10025

WORK (212) 960-2137
HOME (212) 496-4142

OBJECTIVE
HOSPITAL ADMINISTRATOR
Managerial/administrative position at the departmental level or in core administration

SUMMARY
M.P.A. degree and four years' experience in health care administration. Prepare and review budgets up to $500,000. Adept at troubleshooting and formulating systems to solve operational problems. Extensive personnel experience, including ability to supervise, motivate, and counsel employees.

HEALTH CARE ADMINISTRATION EXPERIENCE

1986–present
ST. JOSEPH'S HOSPITAL CENTER, New York, New York
Administrative Manager, Emergency Services Department (1979–present)
Administer all aspects of Emergency Department, including line supervision of clerical staff of 21. Prepare budget and review expenditures, formulate and interpret departmental policies for all personnel; purchase and maintain equipment, oversee M.D. staffing of Screening Clinic.
- Reduced projected overtime requirements by 40% annually through institution of relief position with staggered hours; cut overtime costs and improved staff morale
- Department came within budget in 1987 for first time in three years, owing to careful budget preparation based on actual spending adjusted for projected growth and inflation, monthly review of expenditures, and investigation of unusual expenses
- Upgraded levels of supervisory personnel in order to clarify lines of authority and improve accountability for clerical performance
- Conceived and implemented weekly multidisciplinary conference for review of problems and recommendation of appropriate actions, significantly improving both communication and staff cooperation

1985–1986
MONTESSORI HOSPITAL AND MEDICAL CENTER OF BROOKLYN, Brooklyn, New York
Manager, Personnel Grants
Organized and administered operations of CETA on-the-job training program for 34 employees, including orientation, counseling, and partial supervision; ensured conformity to governmental regulations and effective liaison with outside agencies; initiated and maintained all data systems
- Hospital grossed more than $65,000 in nine months, owing to careful program implementation and monitoring
- Compiled and wrote CETA manual, clarified and systematized hospital's responsibilities for participation and reimbursement, and provided continuity for program administration
- Participated in personnel employment and wage/salary activities—for instance, communicated with union hiring hall, screened applicants, conducted salary surveys, and wrote jobs descriptions

THELMA L. CUMMINGS
PAGE 2

1985 NEW YORK HOSPITAL, New York, New York
Administrative Resident
Rotated through hospital departments, line responsibility as Administrator-on-Call, completed special projects as assigned
- Successfully coordinated and collected Medicaid and Blue Cross surveys required for reimbursement in one-twelfth normal time; resulted in recommendation for employment at MHMCB
- Proposed systematization of photocopying operations and equipment for projected savings of 30%; data generated from this study was used to help equip new hospital under construction

BUSINESS AND PUBLIC SERVICE EXPERIENCE

1985 DAVID DONLAN FOR COUNTY EXECUTIVE (political campaign), Garden City, New York
Office Manager/Bookkeeper
Set up systems for cash flow and fiscal operations, prepared financial statements for submission to Board of Elections, and arranged meetings with community and political leaders

1983 PILOT FABRICS CORPORATION, New York, New York
Assistant Convertor/Shipping Supervisor
Assisted in directing conversion of raw goods to finished textiles; served as liaison and troubleshooter to ensure on-schedule activity of mills, dyers, and truckers; and maintained effective communications with customers

1980–1981 UNITED WAY OF GREATER NEW YORK, New York, New York
Fund-Raiser
Organized and assisted campaign committees and groups; arranged promotional, educational, and fund-raising events

EDUCATION NEW YORK UNIVERSITY, GRADUATE SCHOOL OF PUBLIC ADMINISTRATION, New York, New York
    1985—M.P.A., Health Policy, Planning and Administration (4.0 cumulative average)
NEW YORK UNIVERSITY, WASHINGTON SQUARE COLLEGE, New York, New York.
    1979—B.A., Religion (Founders' Day Honors Certificate; 3.9 cumulative average)
VASSAR COLLEGE, Poughkeepsie, New York
    1974–976—64 credits toward B.S., Religion and Biology (Dean's List)
Additional Professional Study:
    1986—Grants Writing Seminar, North Group of Falls Church, Virginia
    1982—Group Dynamics in Human Relations, New School for Social Research

AFFILIATIONS American Public Health Association
American Hospital Association

MANAGED CARE MARKETING EXECUTIVE

JOAN LARSON
427 Jefferson Street
Geneva, Illinois 60134
(630) 232-2871

SUMMARY

Highly effective and creative leader with 20 years of sales and marketing experience in managed care. Skilled communicator with ability to relate complex services and programs to all levels of management and employees. Self-starter with ability to work well independently and as team leader. Insight into successful entrepreneurial ventures and sustaining sales in high growth industries.

PROFESSIONAL EXPERIENCE

HEALTHCO CONTAINMENT SERVICES, INC., Shaumburg, Illinois   1987–1995
Prescription Benefit Manager with over $7 billion of client drug expenditures.
A Division of Miles Laboratories.

<u>Director of Sales</u>
Responsible for prospect qualification, program presentation, proposal customization, program consulting and evaluation, closure of sales, overseeing implementation, and contract negotiation.
- Established midwestern office and territory.
- Created business opportunities and long term relationships with Fortune 150 companies, Blue Cross-Blue Shield Plans, Health Maintenance Organizations and Unions.
- Developed long term partnerships with Insurance Companies, Healthcare Consultants, and Third Party Administrators to educate and provide prescription benefit services for their clients.
- Cultivated and participated in sale of Central States Teamsters Health and Welfare Fund with over 160,000 active members and 140,000 annuitants which resulted in over $80 million of annual client drug expenditure.
- Closed sales with major corporations: Commonwealth Edison, Honeywell, American National Can, Anheuser-Busch Companies, Johnson Controls, Fortis Insurance Company, A.G. Edwards, AO Smith, which represented over 200,000 eligible employees and retirees and over $70 million of annual client drug expenditures.

PARTNERS NATIONAL HEALTH PLANS, Park Ridge, Illinois   1985–1987
Joint venture created by Voluntary Hospitals of America (VHA) and Aetna Life Insurance Company to develop and manage preferred provider products and health maintenance organizations.

<u>Marketing Director</u>
Responsible for the development of marketing plans, local marketing materials, advertising strategies, and sales strategies for service areas including Chicago, Milwaukee, Indianapolis, and Rockford.
- Identified hospitals for a marketable PPO Network.
- Served as liaison between corporate marketing, network hospitals, and Aetna sales personnel.
- Trained and assisted Aetna with sales presentation of managed care products and programs.
- Acted as Marketing Director for start-up phase of Partners Health Plan of Indiana. Developed and implemented marketing plan, created marketing materials, hired and trained sales team.

JOAN LARSON
Page 2

PERK HEALTH PLAN, Hannibal, Missouri   1983–1985
Federally Qualified Health Maintenance Organization and Preferred Provider Organization.

<u>Marketing Director</u>
Responsible for direction and supervision of Sales and Account Management departments, development of annual market plans, budgets and direction of advertising campaigns. Enrollment increased 30 percent from 26,000 members to 37,000 members.

MICHAEL REESE HEALTH PLAN, Chicago, Illinois   1980–1983
<u>Sales Manager</u>

NORTH SHORE HEALTH PLAN, INC., Glencoe, Illinois   1978–1980
<u>Marketing Representative</u>

EDUCATIONAL BACKGROUND

Master in Public Health, 1977
Health Resource Management
University of Illinois,
Chicago Medical Center Campus,
Chicago, Illinois

B.A. History, 1973
University of Illinois,
Champaign, Illinois

Northern Illinois University, 1969–1971
Dekalb, Illinois

NURSE EXECUTIVE

Timothy Ruschel • 1876 Campbell Street • Athens, Georgia 30605 • (404) 781-4617

Employed by Healthcare Organizations since 1983 with increasingly responsible positions managing hospital services.

EXPERIENCE

ATHENS REGIONAL HOSPITAL, Athens, Georgia   1989-1994
105-bed Sole Community Hospital

Senior Vice President / Chief Operating Officer
Administration of all support departments, ancillary departments, surgery areas, and primary care outreach program. Accountability and responsibility for 200 FTEs and $18 million annual operating expenses.

- Developed or acquired five primary care practices; obtained Rural Health Clinic Status for several; recruitment of physicians and nurse practitioners for primary care services to preserve community vitality and capture enrollment under managed care.
- Design of new facility with relocation.
- Technology assessment and management (cardiac cath lab, echo, mobile MR, mobile lithotripsy, CT, tunable dye laser).
- Directed successful JCAHO surveys in 1993 and 1990; negotiated with and guided application process, increasing annual net income almost $4 million over three years.
- Department redesign, reducing expense and improving quality.
- Guided capital projects through Georgia CN process.
- Directed OSHA and CLIA compliance activities.
- Wrote weekly newspaper column bonding hospital and community.

AMI-AUGUSTA REGIONAL HOSPITAL, Augusta, Georgia   1988-1989
301-bed Investor-owned Hospital

Marketing Administrator, 1989
Administration of marketing and public relations, laboratory, and pharmacy; accountability and responsibility for 60 employees and $4 million annual operating expense.

- Developed marketing database, tracking interaction of population, referring physicians and hospital services.
- Developed physician liaison program, physician outreach services, Directory.
- Launched fundamental hospital redirection focused on care of elderly with integrated clinical psychiatric program.
- Wrote TV, radio, billboard, and print ads.

Administrative Resident, 1988
Revised hospital chargemaster, examined clinical program feasibility, participated in joint venture negotiation and performed physician practice valuation.

Timothy Ruschel • Page 2

LINCOLN VETERANS HOSPITAL, Augusta, Georgia   1983–1989
334-bed Teaching Hospital

Registered Nurse
Coronary care, intensive care, surgery units; direct mail recruitment letters, print ads; redesigned service delivery system for telemetry; modeled costs of telemetry waiting and staff turnover; shift supervision; developed, wrote, and edited staff newsletter.

EDUCATION

Master of Science in Public Health / Health Services Management (MHA)   1988
University of Georgia - Athens, Georgia
  Designed TQM program for University Hospital Clinics (170,000 visits/year); examined patient physician and information flow, internal quality; designed monitors; redesigned systems to become fail-safe; initiated staff training.

Associate of Science - Nursing   1983
Georgia Southwestern College, Americus, Georgia
  Graduated cum laude

Bachelor of Journalism (News-Editorial)   1977
University of Georgia - Athens, Georgia
  Graduated cum laude

LICENSURE/AFFILIATIONS

Affiliate, American College of Healthcare Executives   1989

Georgia Licensed Registered Nurse, 1983; ACLS   1990

COMMUNITY ACTIVITIES

Sponsor and Advisor, Medical Explorers Post

Member, Advisory Board, Athens Area Vocational-Technical School

MISCELLANEOUS ELECTRONIC RÉSUMÉS

The electronically generated résumés reprinted on the following pages appear essentially as they were downloaded from the computer from three online job-search sources. All names and addresses have been removed, however, and most obvious errors have been corrected. Suggestions for other specific entry improvements appear in the margins.

As you go through these résumés, decide—based on advice given earlier in the chapter—what additional design or word changes would make your résumé more communicative or appealing than the samples included. When using many online job-search services, you won't have the option of adjusting the type size of your résumé, for example, or of using boldface, italics, or underlining for emphasis. Your only alternative may be to make creative use of white space to improve readability, such as through vertical and horizontal spacing.

Suggestion: Print out your résumé after inputting the personal and professional data asked for, to see what a prospective employer will see. If the overall impact falls short of your expectations (ask one or more trusted colleagues for ideas), make all appropriate changes and corrections and try again.

ACUTE CARE NURSE

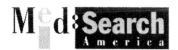

Acute Care Nurse
Applicant Code: ◄—— *MedSearch America identifies members with an Applicant Code number,*
Occupation: *Nursing*   *rather than by name, address, and phone number.*
Desired Work Status: *Full-Time*
Primary Job Location: *San Bernardino, CA*
Relocation City: *Nashville, TN; Bozeman, MT; Hartford, CT*
Relocation Country: *Norway*

PROFESSIONAL OBJECTIVE:	Seeking entrance level RN position, acute care
EXPERIENCE:	
10/95 to 01/96	Bellaire Residence, Home Health RN Loma Linda, CA Care-planning, catheterization ◄—— *Transpose these two entries to assure consistent reverse chronological sequence.*
10/95 to Present	Skills Lab Instructor Loma Linda University School of Nursing
03/94 to 06/94	Practicum: Emergency Room Loma Linda Medical Center Triage, pediatrics, cardiac, trauma, respiratory
06/92 to 09/92	Vintage Faire Convalescent Hospital, CNA Modesto, CA V/S, I&O's, ADL's, colostomy care
06/90 to 12/91	Oak Valley Care Center, CNA Oakdale, CA V/S, I&O's, ADL's, colostomy care
EDUCATION:	
09/92 to 06/95	Loma Linda University Bachelor of Science in Nursing
09/91 to 06/92	Pacific Union College, Angwin, CA Prerequisites for nursing.
09/90 to 06/91	Newbold College, Bracknell, England Prerequisites for nursing.
CERTIFICATIONS:	BLS-C expires 10/09/96, ACLS expires 12/97 applied for PHN 01/96
ACTIVITIES:	
09/93 to Present	Leader for Children's Hospital Ministry Loma Linda Medical Center Azure Hills Kid's Konnection church program
09/92 to 06/94	School of Nursing Representative for Collegiate Advocates for Better Living
09/86 to Present	Homeless feeding projects, Medical Mission trips to Mexico, church's Pathfinder Club

INTERESTS: Back-packing, jogging, mountain-biking, music, volleyball

Date Submitted: 02/05/96 ⬅ **Date downloaded from computer**

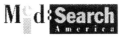 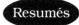 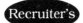

Copyright © 1994–1996 MedSearch America, Inc.
Send feedback to MedSearch America.

SOCIAL WORKER

CERTIFIED SOCIAL WORKER

All candidate names, addresses, and phone numbers have been deleted.

OBJECTIVE:
To find a suitable position as a Certified Social Worker, preferably in North Carolina or Arizona. Other areas are open for consideration.

EDUCATION:
FORDHAM UNIVERSITY, Graduate School of Social Services, Tarrytown, NY
Master's Degree in Social Work May 1986
Major: Services to Individuals and Families

MARIST COLLEGE, Poughkeepsie, NY
Bachelor's Degree in Social Work May 1985 Cum Laude

DUTCHESS COMMUNITY COLLEGE, Poughkeepsie, NY
Associate's Degree in Applied Science May 1983
Major: Community Mental Health Assistant

CERTIFICATION:
Credential Alcoholism Counselor July 1993
Certified Social Worker November 1986

EXPERIENCE:
10/93–Present ST. FRANCIS HOSPITAL, TURNING POINT, Admissions Dept., Beacon, NY

Assess appropriateness of persons interested in admission, offer clinical feedback to coworkers, facilitate admissions to detox and rehab, and present new cases at daily interdisciplinary treatment planning meeting.

4/91–10/93 ST. FRANCIS HOSPITAL, TURNING POINT, Beacon, NY
Supervision of alcoholism counselors, completing employee evaluations, facilitating group therapy, family interventions, individual counseling, and discharge planning in 30-bed detoxification unit.

1986–1991 ST. FRANCIS HOSPITAL, Poughkeepsie, NY
Developed safe aftercare plans for patients of all ages, provided appropriate psycho-social information when necessary to facilitate transfers, worked with various community agencies to assist patients in obtaining appropriate services, trained HIV/AIDS counselors, certified in pre- and post-test counseling.

INTERNSHIP:
1985–1986 VASSAR BROTHERS HOSPITAL, Social Service Dept., Poughkeepsie, NY
Primary focus was discharge planning and facilitating a diabetic support group.

1983–1985 DUTCHESS OUTREACH, Poughkeepsie, NY
Interviewed and assessed client needs and provided emergency food and clothing.

HUDSON RIVER PSYCHIATRIC CENTER, Poughkeepsie, NY
Participated in treatment planning, co-facilitating groups, and charted documentation in an all male ward for chronic psychiatric patients.

1981–1983 BOCES, Salt Point, NY
Worked with children with varying degrees of emotional and developmental disabilities.

CONTINUING SERVICE CENTER, Poughkeepsie, NY
Directly involved in educational programs geared to enhance ADL skills.

CEREBRAL PALSY REHABILITATION CLINIC, Poughkeepsie, NY
Worked with children with severe physical and mental handicaps.

HYDE PARK NURSING HOME, Hyde Park, NY
Assisted patients with transition, wrote psycho-social assessments, participated in treatment planning, and counseled family members with ongoing difficulty placing family members in a nursing home.

Identifies online service, and date résumé was downloaded.

2-11-1996 America Online:Indexking Page 1

CRITICAL CARE NURSE

CRITICAL CARE OR EMERGENCY DEPARTMENT STAFF RN

JOB TARGET:
Critical Care or Emergency Department Staff RN (Adult or Pediatric) with flexibility in considering other areas of nursing.

KEY WORDS:
RN, BA, ACLS, PALS, PALS Instructor, BCLS Instructor, Emergency, 4 years' experience, Pediatrics, and diverse population.

CAPABILITIES:
* ACLS (Advanced Cardiac Life Support) Provider (7/94).
* PALS (Pediatric Advanced Life Support) Provider (5/93) and Instructor (3/95).
* BCLS (Basic Cardiac Life Support) Provider (3/85) and Instructor (9/92).
* Nationally Registered and Minnesota Licensed EMT-A (5/91).
* Work effectively with a culturally diverse population.
* Work in an effective and orderly fashion.
* Communicate effectively with patients and staff.
* Flexible in meeting patient and unit needs.
* Manage time well.
* Well versed in many emergency procedures (Ingestion management, splinting, bandaging, bleeding control, fracture reduction, cervical spine immobilization and triage.)
* Computer literate.

ACCOMPLISHMENTS:
* Received Anoka County Voiture 40 et 8 nursing scholarship.
* Dean's List at UMM and ARCC.
* UMM Freshman Academic Scholar.
* Historian of the Chi Phi Fraternity.
* Secretary/Treasurer of the UMM Juggling Club.
* Anoka Youth Salute recipient.
* Graduated with honors from Anoka Senior High School.

ACTIVITIES:
* Teaching for the PALS course offered by the Medical Education Department at Children's Health Care-Minneapolis since 7/93.
* Teaching for the BCLS recertification course at Children's Health Care-Minneapolis since 9/92.
* Presented in a break out session on pediatric trauma care at the American Heart Association "Toward Total Life Support" conference in St. Cloud, MN on 2/25/95.

WORK EXPERIENCE:
* EMT (Emergency Medical Technician) in the Emergency Department at Children's Health Care, Minneapolis. Also occasionally functioned as a Health Unit Coordinator. 1991 to present.
* Vehicle Emissions Inspector at Envirotest Technologies Inc. 1992 to 1993
* Teaching Assistant in Psychology Department at the University of Minnesota, Morris. 1991 academic year
* Server at Perkin's Family Restaurant in Anoka, Minnesota. 1986 to 1989
* Seasonal Factory Laborer at Longview Fibre Company in Fridley, Minnesota. 1988 to 1989

EDUCATION:
* Associate of Science in Nursing. June, 1995. Anoka-Ramsey Community College. Coon Rapids, Minnesota.
* Bachelor of Arts in Psychology (minor in Biology). 1991, University of Minnesota, Morris.

References available upon request

Transmitted: 95-03-22 17:01:19 EST

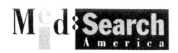

MA Exercise Science/Cardiac Rehab
Applicant Code:
Occupation: *Dietetics/Nutrition/Fitness*
Desired Work Status: *Full-Time*
Relocation City: *Virginia, Maryland, Delaware*

EDUCATION

Master of Arts — University of Georgia — December 1995 ◄ *Should consider (1) combining "Honors/Memberships" as part of the Education section; and/or (2) placing Education at the end of the résumé, placing his powerful Work Experience first.*
Exercise Science

Bachelor of Science — State University of New York College at Cortland — December 1992
Physical Education
(Adult Fitness)

Associate of Applied Science — Penn State University — August 1989
Telecommunications Technology

WORK EXPERIENCE

Laboratory Technician III
The Clinical and Sports Nutrition Laboratory
The University of Georgia, Athens, GA
November 1994–present
* Order all supplies and maintain an adequate inventory.
* Assist in the preparation of manuscripts for publication in scientific journals.
* Assess body composition using a dual-energy X-ray absorptiometer (DEXA).
* Responsible for recruiting and scheduling subjects for research projects.

Personal Fitness Trainer
The Georgia Rehabilitation and Fitness Center, Athens, GA
May 1995–present
* Design and implement individualized fitness programs.

Graduate Teaching Assistant
The University of Georgia, Athens, GA
September 1992–June 1994
* Instructed undergraduate fitness/wellness courses.
* Developed lesson plans and lectured on various health related issues.

Intern (Phase II Cardiac Rehabilitation/Adult Fitness)
The Thomas P. Saxton Pavilion, Wilkes-Barre, PA Summer 1992
* Assisted in developing exercise programs for cardiac rehabilitation patients.
* Monitored heart rate and blood pressure during exercise.
* Lead warm-up and cool-down activities.

Weight Training Instructor
YMCA, Pittston, PA
Summer 1992
* Created and supervised a weight training program for adolescents.

Assistant Manager
The Dough Company, Wilkes-Barre, PA
June 1987–September 1989
* Responsible for the day-to-day operation of an Italian restaurant with a 150 person seating capacity.
* Managed 10–15 employees per shift.

PRESENTATIONS/PUBLICATIONS
* Estimates of Body Composition Using a Four-Component Model in Men with High Musculoskeletal Development: Poster presentation—FASEB 1995.
* Density of the Fat-Free Mass and Body Composition Estimates in Weight Trainers: Submitted for publication in Journal of Applied Physiology.

HONORS/MEMBERSHIPS
* Dean's List: State University of New York College at Cortland—Fall 90, 91
* Kunkle Academic Scholarship: Penn State University—Spring 1987
* Member: American College of Sports Medicine
* Kunkle Academic Scholarship: Pennsylvania State University—Spring 1987
* Member: American College of Sports Medicine

COMPUTER SKILLS
IBM
* Word Perfect 5.1–6.1
* Aldus Persuasion
* Sigmaplot
* Harvard Graphics

Macintosh
* Microsoft Word 5.1–6.01
* Microsoft Excel 4.0–5.0
* Cricket Graph
* Systat 5.2.1
* Pegasus Mail

References available upon request.

Date Submitted: 09/20/95

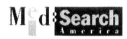 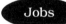 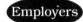 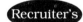

Copyright © 1994–1996 MedSearch America, Inc.
Send feedback to MedSearch America.

LABORATORY TECHNICIAN

LABORATORY POSITION HEALTHCARE/BIOTECHNOLOGY

KEYWORDS:
Bachelor of Science. Biology. Microbiology. Chemistry. Business. Computers. IBM. Word. Minitab. Interpersonal and Communication Skills. Detail Oriented. Reliable. Strong Work Ethic. Laboratory Skills.

OBJECTIVE:
A laboratory position in the healthcare/biotechnology industry with opportunity for professional growth into sales.

HIGHLIGHTS:
Background in biology, chemistry, and business.
Excellent interpersonal and communication skills.
Analytical and detail oriented.
Works well independently or in team situations.

EDUCATION:
Bachelor of Science, Virginia Tech. Blacksburg, Virginia. 1996.
Major: Biology. — Minor: Chemistry.
Option: Business. — QCA: 3.1 in major.

LABORATORY SKILLS:
Pour Plating
Spread Plating
Petrifilm
Api Strip
Incubation Plates
Stomacher
Dilution Schemes
Tube Inoculation
Pipeting
Gram Staining
Anerobe Jar
Spectrometer

EMPLOYMENT:
Summer Temporary, Volt Temporary Services. Manassas, Virginia. Summer, 1994.
Assigned to work at a food distribution center for area wholesalers in the Northern Virginia area. Learned to interact successfully with a variety of individuals. Completed all assignments in efficient and timely manner. Assisted at an engineering company that sanitized equipment utilized in pasteurization processes. Work effectively as part of a team.
Construction Laborer, Lewis Construction Company. Manassas, Virginia. Summer, 1993.
Assisted a new contractor completing projects at a major housing development.Completed a variety of manual tasks, learned construction techniques/tools, and developed respect for hard work.

ACTIVITIES:
Virginia Tech Weight Club.
Intramural Sports.

This resume was prepared for upload by:
OnLine Solutions, Inc.
1584 Rt22B
Morrisonville, NY 12962
Voice: 518-643-2873
Fax: 518-643-0321 or 518-643-0134
Internet: careerprol@aol.com, careerw@usa.net or
http://crm21.com/
Career and Resume Management - 21st Century!

Transmitted: 95-09-27 06:58:38 EDT

A strong entry-level résumé, calling upon all relevant skills, education, and career-related accomplishments.

MANAGEMENT—MEDICAL INSTRUMENTATION

OPERATIONS SUPERVISOR, QUALITY ASSURANCE MANAGER, SERVICE ENGINEER SPECIALIST, MEDICAL TECHNOLOGIST SUPERVISOR, QUALITY CONTROL SUPERVISOR.

SUMMARY:
Results-oriented professional with operations, customer service, and management experience in small to large-sized companies.

Supervising: operations; budgeting and forecasting; employee development; customer support; plant remodeling; materials management, maintaining ISO 9002.

Excellent interpersonal skills, team player and ability to work well with all levels of an organization. Effective presentation, verbal and written communication skills. Well-developed organizational, project management, trouble-shooting and problem-solving abilities, especially related to customer satisfaction.

Computer literate. Proficient in WordPerfect 5.1, Microsoft Excel, Harvard Graphics, Lotus 1-2-3, Microsoft Windows 3.1, DOS 6.2. Familiar with Internet, America On-Line, and Prodigy.
Abilities include: word processing, preparing spreadsheets, flow charting, graphical data analysis.

B.A., University of California at Northridge, CA, Biological Sciences, 1971.

CAREER HISTORY:
1994–present
REPAIR SUPERVISOR, E.I. DuPont World Parts Center, Atlanta, GA. One of the largest medical equipment manufacturers, with revenues of over $850 million and over 5000 employees.

Supervise 18 employees in medical instrument reconditioning; employee development, customer satisfaction, budgeting and forecasting.

Developed new instrument repair/reconditioning process in 1994. Currently program has generated the highest install quality ratings in last four years, savings of new program at $400,000 per year.

Managed $4.4 million budget. Achieved a 20% under P.O. for 1994.

Implement customer call-back program on newly installed instruments. Combined with TQM principles dramatically reduced instrument defects and increased customer satisfaction.

Designed and supervised the construction of 5000 square feet of repair area with a budget of $250,000.

1992–1994
QUALITY CONTROL SUPERVISOR, E.I. DuPont Medical Products Division, Atlanta, GA. A repair/distribution site for medical parts and equipment.

Supervised 17 employees in quality control, employee development, warehouse receiving, supplier returns, budgeting and forecasting.

Streamlined operations by transferring receiving responsibility to general warehouse operations.

Integrated return/used parts inspection to repair operations, resulting in reduction of personnel and more efficient process flow.

Instigated new inspection sampling criteria, resulting in 10% decrease in workload. Directed ISO 9002 certification.

1985–1992
FIELD SERVICE ENGINEER, E.I. DuPont Medical Products Division, Atlanta, GA. Equipment service and support organization for DuPont's diagnostic medical equipment.

Achieved and maintained a $350,000 customer contract base. Increased revenue due to removal of all third party service competition.

Designed a national marketing package, illustrating the current product line.

Responsible for generating sales of over $3 million.

Created multi-business communication network that led to increased business and customer satisfaction.

Organized and conducted numerous customer training workshops, which resulted in fewer repair calls.

Facilitator for Xerox's customer satisfaction course. Taught field service engineers interaction skills.

1984–1985
FIELD SERVICE ENGINEER, Labtronics, Inc., Palo Alto, CA. A third party service company repairing medical laboratory equipment.

Developed new equipment processes that added $50,000/yr. in new revenues.

Outsourced service parts to save over 50% on current pricing.

1983–1984
CLINICAL LABORATORY SUPERVISOR, Pathology Laboratories, Los Gatos, CA.

Supervised four employees in analysis of clinical laboratory specimens for hematology, urinalysis, coagulation, serology.

1981–1983
QUALITY CONTROL MANAGER, Advanced Technical Services, Fremont, CA. Company providing circuit board assembly.

Supervision of 32 employees involved with inspection of circuit boards.

Developed department from 10 employees to 32 employees in 1.5 years.

1973–1981
SENIOR MEDICAL TECHNOLOGIST, Los Gatos Community Hospital, Los Gatos, CA.

Performed analysis on clinical specimens.

Directed special chemistry department. Revised over 50% of procedures, resulting in 20% labor savings.

CERTIFICATION:
Electronics technician
Defensive driving
Hazardous driving conditions

ADDITIONAL TRAINING CLASSES:
First line supervisor
Strategic selling
Helping others succeed
Customer satisfaction
ISO/GMP
Sexual harassment issues
Diversity

Transmitted: 95-08-18 11:41:08 EDT

Well-worded, accomplishments-oriented Career History entries; Summary serves as effective introduction. Problem areas: (1) A "dense" appearance may turn off some readers. Should consider cutting less important entries, and adding vertical space between entries to improve readability. (2) Too many objectives listed at top of first page. Candidate would be better off concentrating on one Objective per résumé, with all subsequent entries related to that Objective. Fewer words will also improve readability.

MEDICAL ASSISTANT

Subject: Résumé: Medical Assistant
From:
Date Posted: 9 Jan 1996 19:32:17 GMT
Organization: (none specified)
Newsgroups: misc.jobs.resumes, us.jobs.resumes

Name:
Company: (none specified)
E-mail:
Phone:
Location: Syracuse and Suburbs

OBJECTIVE: To obtain a position in the health care industry utilizing my medical assisting skills

EDUCATION: BRYANT & STRATTON BUSINESS INSTITUTE
    Syracuse, NY. Associate in Occupational Studies
    Major: Medical Assisting. 1994–1995
  ONONDAGA MEDICAL CAREER SCHOOL
    Syracuse, NY. Medical Transcription. June–August 1993
  CENTRAL CITY BUSINESS INSTITUTE
    Syracuse, NY. Associate in Occupational Studies
    Major: Medical Administrative Studies. 1988–1990

SKILLS:
  CLINICAL
    Knowledge of a variety of testing/operational procedures including: operation of an autoclave, recording electrocardiograms, performing capillary punctures/phlebotomy, able to assist with physical exams/minor surgery, proficient with injections, fixing/gram staining a specimen slide.
  CLERICAL
    Word processing: WordPerfect, Professional Write, Microsoft Word 6.0, spreadsheets, database.
    Transcription: Medical dictation 40wpm, schedule appointments, record patient's history, telephone skills, microfilm.

WORK EXPERIENCE:
  INTERNSHIP
    North Medical Family Physicians, Liverpool, NY.
    Clinical/Clerical duties. (June–August 1995)
  MEDICAL ASSISTANT
    Robert S. Phillips, M.D., P.C., Gynecologist, Syracuse, NY.
    Responsibilities: Took and recorded BP/height/weight/test results, tested urine samples, sterilized instruments, cleaned and prepared rooms. (On call December 1993–June 1994)
  VOLUNTEER
    Plaza Health and Rehabilitation Center, Syracuse, NY.
    Developed effective phone skills as a receptionist for Physical Therapy Department. Transported patients. (December 1993–February 1994)
  VOLUNTEER
    St. Joseph's Hospital Health Center, Syracuse, NY.
    Performed various tasks around the hospital (July–August 1993)

CURRENT CERTIFICATIONS:
CPR/First Aid

MEDICAL TECHNOLOGIST

MEDICAL OR RESEARCH TECHNOLOGIST—ASCP, NCA

CAREER OBJECTIVES:
Employment as a Medical or Research Technologist for a Biotechnology Company or Hospital

EDUCATION:
New York Methodist Hospital, Brooklyn, NY
School of Medical Technology
August, 1994–August, 1995
Award for Excellence in Blood Banking
Award for Excellence in Clinical Biochemistry
Award for Overall Excellence in Clinical Pathology

Bates College, Lewiston, ME
BS Biology, May 1985
Dean's List, 1985

Carnegie-Mellon University, Pittsburgh, PA
1981–1983
Dean's List, 1981

WORK EXPERIENCE:
Medical Technologist, Debrah Hammond, Lab Director
Pecos County Memorial Hospital
Sanderson Highway, Fort Stockton, TX 79735
October 2, 1995–present

Medical Technologist, Carol Staples, Lab Director
New York Methodist Hospital
506 Sixth St., Brooklyn, NY 11215–9008
March 6, 1995–September 22, 1995

Administrative Assistant/Receptionist
Vanguard Temporaries, Inc.
211 East 43rd St., New York, NY 10017
June, 1994–August, 1994

Research Technician, Dr. George Happ
Dept. of Zoology, Univ. of Vermont, Burlington, VT 05406
August, 1991–April, 1994

Research Technician, Dr. Judith van Houten
Dept. of Zoology, Univ. of Vermont
August, 1990–August, 1991

Research Technician
R & D Systems, Inc., Growth Factor Dept.
614 McKinley Place NE, Minneapolis, MN 55413
September, 1989–June, 1990

Senior Laboratory Technician, Dr. Larry Lasky
Dept. of Lab Medicine and Pathology, Univ. of Minnesota
May, 1989–September, 1989

Senior Laboratory Technician, Dr. S.M.N. Efange
Dept. of Radiology, Univ. of Minnesota
August, 1988–May, 1989

Research Assistant, Dr. Thomas Dick

(1) As a newly graduated technologist, candidate's Education is properly listed first. (2) For a more forceful presentation, job responsibilities and accomplishments should be added to each of the Work Experience entries. (3) The "Research Assistant" entry (bottom of résumé) needs a reference point to give it relevance.

2-11-1996 America Online:Indexking Page 1

MEDICAL SALES/MARKETING MANAGEMENT

OBJECTIVE:
Medical Sales / Marketing Management

SUMMARY OF QUALIFICATIONS:
* Professional individual with a strong commitment to a career in the medical industry.
* Over 18 years' sales, marketing and management experience in the medical industry.
* Strong background in sales administration, personnel, sales & marketing.
* Traveling large sales territories; developing strong account relationships.
* Excellent interpersonal and communication skills.
* Strong organization and time management skills.
* Considered self-motivated, people-oriented, a problem solver, and enthusiastic.

PROFESSIONAL EXPERIENCE:
CYTOGEN CORPORATION, Princeton, NJ. August 1992–Present
Special Accounts Manager/Nuclear Oncology Specialist (January 1994–Present)
Territory Manager (August 1992–January 1994)
Presented cost benefit savings data affecting cost and patient management to top administrators of a large buying group. Performed customer training, sales and marketing for the first FDA approved monoclonal antibody for diagnostic imaging of colorectal or recurrent ovarian adenocarcinoma. Called on Nuclear Medicine, Radiology, Oncology, Surgery and Gynecology Departments and Physicians located in Texas and parts of Oklahoma.
Accomplishments:
* Achieved #1 in sales for 1994 in Western United States and #3 nationally.

BRISTOL-MYERS SQUIBB, Princeton, NJ. April 1990–August 1992
Nuclear Medicine Technical Associate
Responsibilities include sales and sales support for Diagnostic Nuclear Medicine products to key accounts and influentials. Provided marketing and competitive information to management. Participated in promotional and sales activities related to Diagnostic Nuclear Medicine. Educated and trained customers for existing and new nuclear medicine products. Organized speakers' programs. Convention coverage. Responsible for South Central Region including portions of Texas, Oklahoma, Louisiana and Mississippi.
Accomplishments:
* 1991 Western Zone winner CardioTec Sales Training contest with highest number of accounts trained to use product.
* Ranked #1 in the nation in 1990 Nuclear Medicine sales.
* 1990 National winner Syncor Pharmacy Sales contest with largest dollar and percent increase.

PARKE DAVIS, Morris Plains, NJ. August 1989–March 1990
Medical Service Representative
Promoted and sold cardiovascular products to cardiologist and internal medicine physicians, as well as seizure control products to neurologists. Presented educational programs on preventing coronary risk non drug and drug therapy and patient and physician educational programs on epilepsy and controlling seizures. Scheduled speakers for hospitals, AMA and AOA functions for cardiovascular and seizure control products.

MOBIL TECHNOLOGY CORP., New York, NY. September 1988–May 1989
Marketing Executive
Sold and marketed high dollar, state-of-the-art medical imaging equipment, MRI, CT and Lithotripters. Assisted in trade show representation covering a five state region.

ABBOTT LABORATORIES, North Chicago, IL. November 1983–September 1988
Professional Medical Representative
Promoted and sold pharmaceutical products, diagnostic lab tests and lab equipment to physicians, pharmacies, labs and hospitals.
Accomplishments:
* Ranked in top 10% of sales force in 1985, 1986 and 1987.
* #1 dollar producer in Southwest Region in key products and a member of Abbott's All-star Team in 1986 and 1987.

DALLAS-FORT WORTH MEDICAL CENTER, Grand Prairie, TX. September 1975–November 1983
Director of Nuclear Medicine
Administrative position responsible for producing over $500,000 revenue per year. Prepared budgets, purchasing requests, patient records and departmental charges. Operated medical computers and gamma camera. Injected radioactive isotopes and monitored quality control. Responsible for education and training of all departmental employees.

EDUCATION:
EAST TEXAS STATE, Commerce, TX
B.S., Health Care Administration

PROFESSIONAL:
CTMN Nuclear Medicine
ARRT in Nuclear Medicine
ARRT in X-Ray
MRI Training

SPECIAL TRAINING:
Specialized Training in Managed Health Care
Xerox Sales Course
Zig Ziglar's Richer Life Course
SMI's Success Motivational Course
Better Business Writing
Building a Business Vocabulary

AFFILIATIONS AND ORGANIZATIONS:
Society of Nuclear Medicine
North Texas Society of Nuclear Medicine
Beta Sigma Phi Sorority

Transmitted: 10/24/95 10:01 AM

A good résumé, but some impact is lost because of its crowded appearance. Add space between entries for improved readability.

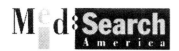

Occupational Therapist
Applicant Code:
Occupation: *Therapy/Rehabilitation*
Desired Work Status: *Full-Time*
Primary Job Location: *Minneapolis, MN*
Relocation City: *St. Paul, MN*

OBJECTIVE:
Occupational Therapist position

EDUCATION:

1993–1995	College of St. Catherine, St. Paul, MN Bachelor of Arts Degree in Occupational Therapy
1977–1979	Anoka Ramsey Community College, Coon Rapids, MN Anoka Hennepin Technical College, Anoka, MN Associate of Arts Degree in Occupational Therapy

CERTIFICATION:
Occupational Therapy Assistant Certification

PROFESSIONAL EXPERIENCE:

Summer 1995   Unity Medical Center
Fridley, MN
Occupational Therapy clinical field work
* Performing acute care evaluation and treatment of orthopedic, neurological, and pulmonary rehabilitation.
* Performing outpatient evaluation and treatment.

Spring 1995   Veterans Administration Medical Center
Minneapolis, MN
Occupational Therapy clinical field work
* Performing standardized functional assessments utilizing the Allen Cognitive Level Test, the Cognitive Performance Test, and the Mini-Mental State Exam.
* Directing the Adapted Work Program—a sheltered workshop for veterans in early to middle stages of dementing disease.
* Supervising COTAs and volunteers.

7/1993–6/1995   Healthspan Homecare and Hospice
Roseville, MN
Certified Occupational Therapy Assistant
* Providing rehabilitative homecare treatment to a variety of diagnoses including CVA and cardiac.
* Developing patient home programs.

PHYSICIAN ASSISTANT

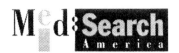

Physician Assistant
Applicant Code:
Occupation: *Physician Assistant*
Desired Work Status: *Full-Time*
Primary Job Location: *Durham, NC*
Relocation City: *Syracuse, NY*

EDUCATION:

1993–Current	Duke University, Physician Assistant Program. Master of Health Science and Physician Assistant certificate to be awarded 1995.
1991–1993 1988–1989	State University of New York at Oswego, Department of Biology/Zoology. Major in Zoology. Bachelor of Arts awarded 1993.
1990–1991	Syracuse University, Department of Biology. Major in Biology. Credits towards Bachelor of Arts.
1989–1990	State University of New York Health Science Center at Upstate Medical Center, Paramedic Program. Paramedic Certificate awarded in 1990.

CLINICAL ROTATIONS:

08/01–08/26/94	Dermatology, Duke University Medical Center. Durham, North Carolina.
08/29–10/24/94	Internal Medicine, Womack Army Hospital. Fayetteville, North Carolina.
10/24–11/18/94	Behavior Medicine, Durham County Substance Abuse Service, Inpatient Treatment Durham Regional Hospital. Durham, North Carolina.
11/21–12/16/94	Pediatrics, All Children's Hospital. St. Petersburg, Florida.
01/03–01/27/95	OB-GYN, Durham Regional Hospital. Durham, North Carolina.
01/30–02/24/95	Research project, Duke University Medical Center. Durham, North Carolina.
03/06–03/31/95	Surgery, Durham Regional Hospital. Durham, North Carolina.
04/03–04/28/95	Orthopedics, Burlington Orthopedics. Burlington, North Carolina.
05/01–05/26/95	Out-patient Medicine, Dr. Ayecock. Mebane, North Carolina.
05/29–06/23/95	Pediatric Infectious Disease, Duke University Medical Center. Durham, North Carolina.
06/26–07/21/95	Emergency Medicine, Duke University Medical Center. Durham, North Carolina.

POSITIONS HELD:

1990–1993	Professional Paramedic Basic and Advanced Life Support care and transport covering the city of Syracuse and surrounding suburbs. Eastern Paramedics. Syracuse, New York.
1991–1993	Professional Paramedic Basic and Advanced Life Support care and transport covering the city of Fulton and Oswego County. Menter Ambulance. Fulton, New York.
1989–1991	Volunteer Emergency Medical Technician Basic Life Support care and transport covering North Syracuse and the town of Clay. North Area Volunteer Ambulance Corporation. North Syracuse, New York.
1988–1990	Volunteer Emergency Medical Technician Basic Life Support care and transport covering Pulaski and Oswego County. Northern Oswego County Ambulance. Pulaski, New York.

PROFESSIONAL AFFILIATIONS:
1993–Current   American Academy of Physician Assistants

1993–Current   North Carolina Academy of Physician Assistants

1993–Current   Stead Society

CREDENTIALS:
Basic Cardiac Life Support
Advanced Cardiac Life Support

PROFESSIONAL OBJECTIVES:
To provide respected and quality healthcare for patients in need. To continue my medical education while pursing a rewarding career as a Physician Assistant.

Date Submitted: 04/24/95

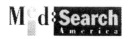 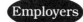 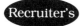

Copyright © 1994–1996 MedSearch America, Inc.
Send feedback to MedSearch America.

Good résumé for entry-level physician assistant, but could do without the detailed dates under "Clinical Rotations."

PSYCHOLOGIST/COUNSELOR

EDUCATION:
1993
Pacifica Graduate Institute, Carpinteria, CA
MA—Counseling Psychology; Specialization in Depth Psychology

1973
University of Arizona, Tucson, AZ
BA—Major: Anthropology; Minor: Philosophy

PROFESSIONAL EXPERIENCE:
1995–1996
Skagit Mental Health Center, Mt. Vernon, WA
MICA Liaison Specialist
Provided liaison services between Skagit Mental Health, the North Sound Regional Support Network agencies, treatment providers and the Pioneer Center North MICA (Mentally Ill Chemically Addicted) program. Promoted referral process between MICA facility and agency of origin. Facilitated resolutions to client grievances with MICA program. Attended weekly staffings, consults with staff and led group and individual therapy sessions.

1990–1995
Southern Arizona Mental Health Center, Tucson, AZ
Mental Health Psychotherapist II
Planned treatment and managed cases of chronically and severely mentally ill individuals as an outreach member of a mobile crisis intervention team. Provided psychiatric evaluation, intervention and follow-up in emergency departments, detention centers, individual's home and community settings. Worked in tandem with law enforcement, adult protective services and other mental health agencies and professionals. Assessed clients for danger to self, others or gravely disabled and/or acutely and persistently disabled. Prepared pre-petition screening reports. Maintained charting and documentation. Witnessed at commitment hearings. Invited to join child emergency team by staff and supervisor and was trained in child and adolescent assessment and crisis intervention

1989
Family Counseling Agency, Tucson, AZ
Case Manager
Provided in-home assessments of older and disabled adults to receive medical services, home health aid, and fitted appliances enabling clients to live independently. Evaluated need for psychotherapy.

1973–1989
Missionaries of Charity
Catholic Religious Brother
Established and headed houses for Catholic religious brothers in ghettoes of Cambodia, Los Angeles and Dominican Republic in order to fulfill Mother Teresa of Calcutta's vow of serving the "poorest of the poor." Also served in Vietnam and Haiti. Provided medical, food and clothing assistance, literacy classes, and ministry to malnourished children, families fleeing political persecution, the homeless, alcoholics and drug abusers. Appointed by congregation as Novice Master, Retreat Director and General Counselor. The latter was part of a four-man administrative team that oversaw the welfare of the 450-member religious order worldwide. Established House of Prayer for congregational and individual retreats in Albuquerque, NM.

1971–1973
Pima County Hospital, Tucson, AZ
Psychiatric Attendant
Assisted medical staff in providing nursing care, basic counseling and documenting progress for in-patients at neuropsychiatric ward.

1969–1971
Intermountain Aviation
Security Guard
Supervised security entrances and radio landing information for large urban airport. Obtained Department of Defense Security Clearance.

PSYCHOLOGIST/COUNSELOR

ADDITIONAL PROFESSIONAL AND PERSONAL INFORMATION:
Advanced Proficiency in Spanish
Southern Arizona Mental Health Center's Employee Recognition Award—1993
Attended Workshops in Process Oriented Psychology—1991–92
Department of Defense Security Clearance—1969
Private Pilot License—1968
Weaver, Hiker, Camper, Avid Reader, Jazz Aficionado

Transmitted: 95-07-10 15:40:00 EDT

Well-worded résumé with good specifics. Entries need to be broken up to improve readability. (Also, candidate's "Specialization" under Education may be confusing, regardless of the school's official title: Is it "Depth Psychology," or "In-Depth Psychology"?

REGISTERED DIETITIAN

REGISTERED DIETITIAN (R.D.)

EMPLOYMENT DESIRED:
Full-time. Food Service Director, Long Term Care; Dietitian, Health Promotion/Wellness Program; Food Service Management; District Manager, Food and Nutrition Services

PROFESSIONAL ACCOMPLISHMENTS:
Devised and expanded nutrition care programs for 700-bed facility.

Developed and controlled $1–3.5 million budget for Hospital Food and Nutrition Services Departments.

Revised the food production program of hospital cafeterias and patient meal services, including menu and standard recipe development, job descriptions, in-service education programs, quality assurance (QA) programs.

Coordinated the evaluation process and purchase of the modernized patient delivery system for the Millard Fillmore Hospitals (downtown and suburban locations).

Planned, designed and implemented all phases of reconstruction of the cafeterias and kitchens at the Buffalo General Hospital and Millard Fillmore Suburban Hospital.

Supervision of 50–150 employees.

Responsible for overseeing and actively participating in numerous catered events for physicians and hospital personnel such as special parties, picnics, luncheons and dinners, varying from 20–800 people.

EDUCATIONAL BACKGROUND:
State University College at Buffalo, NY–1978
BS Clinical Dietetics, Coordinated Undergraduate Program
Cum Laude Graduate
Dean's List (1974–1978)

WORK HISTORY:
Millard Fillmore Suburban Hospital, Williamsville, NY—September, 1989 to December, 1994
Director, Food and Nutrition Services Department

Buffalo General Hospital, Buffalo, NY—1981 to 1989
Nutritional Services Department
Associate Director—November, 1985 to September, 1989
Acting Director—July, 1985 to November, 1985
Associate Director—December, 1982 to July, 1985
Assistant Director, Clinical Services—September, 1981 to December, 1982

Deaconess Hospital, Buffalo, NY—May, 1978 to September, 1981
Division of The Buffalo General Hospital Corporation
Dietary Department
Chief Clinical Dietitian—September, 1980 to September, 1981
Clinical Dietitian—May, 1978 to September, 1980

PROFESSIONAL AFFILIATIONS:
Western New York Dietetic Association
New York Dietetic Association
American Dietetic Association

SPECIAL HONORS:
Recognized Young Dietitian of the Year—1982
American Dietetic Association

First Alternate "Young Career Woman"—1983
Business and Professional Women's Club of Buffalo, NY

COMMUNITY SERVICE:
Selected to serve on the Nutrition Advisory Council of the Dietetics Program at D'Youville College of Buffalo, NY—1993

Developed program to provide hot luncheon meals to Senior Citizen Center in Western New York Community—1992 to present

American Cancer Society Volunteer—1986 to present

Conducted various nutrition lectures for general public and professional groups; numerous presentations on local television and radio programs as well as in schools, libraries and convention centers—1982 to present

Chairmanship of "National Nutrition Month" campaign for Western New York Dietetic Association for 2 years—1980 and 1981.

Organized committee of Western New York Dietitians involved in diabetes teaching to collectively revise diet instructional materials—1979.

March of Dimes Walk-a-Thon—1974 to present.

References available upon request.

SOURCE: DDragan

Transmitted: 95-02-16 19:16:41 EST

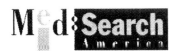

Registered Respiratory Therapist with experience
Applicant Code:
Occupation: *Therapy/Rehabilitation*
Desired Work Status: *Full-Time*
Primary Job Location: *Toronto, Hamilton*
Relocation City: *Pittsburgh, PA; Detroit; MI; Buffalo, NY*
Relocation Country: *USA*

OBJECTIVES:
To further my education and profession while providing quality care for patients of all ages.

EDUCATION:
Registered Respiratory Therapist
Fanshawe College diploma / Canadian Board of Respiratory Care
pass with honours.
1460 Oxford Street, London, Ont.

Bachelor's of Science in Biology
Lake Superior State University
Sault Ste. Marie, MI 49783, USA

Candidate has included no dates for either Education or Work Experience, which will cause many readers to wonder why. Also, the absence of both job responsibilities and accomplishments under Work Experience makes this a weaker section than it need be.

CLINICAL EXPERIENCE:
All in Level III critical care centers.

Diagnostic assessment of patients, neonatal to adult.
Initiation, maintenance and weaning of acute and chronic ventilation.
Advanced hemodynamic and metabolic monitoring.
Pulmonary function, ECG and cardiac stress testing.
OR maintenance and intubation.

WORK EXPERIENCE:
Women's College Hospital. Level III Neonatal and Adult critical care.
76 Grenville Ave., Toronto, Ont.
Casual/Part-time Respiratory Therapist for NICU, ICU, ER
MED/SURG and OR.

MEMBERSHIPS/CERTIFICATIONS:
Member in good standing: College of Respiratory Therapists.
                          Respiratory Therapy Society of Ontario.
                          Canadian Society of Respiratory Therapists.
ACLS, BCLS, Neonatal Resuscitation Practitioner Certified.

References available upon request.

Date Submitted: 03/11/96

SPEECH-LANGUAGE PATHOLOGIST

US - MN, IL, WI - Minneapolis, Chicago, Milwaukee
Speech-Language Pathologist

Candidate Information:
Name:
E-mail:
Street:
City:
State:
Country:
Phone:

Level of Education: MA or MS
Years of Experience: Entry Level

Job Title Desired: Speech-Language Pathologist
Job Location Desired: Minneapolis, Chicago, Milwaukee, MN, IL, WI

Skills for Desired Job: see Résumé

The enthusiastic "Message to the hiring manager" is an innovative and eye-catching way for an entry-level speech-language pathologist to add a personal dimension to—and thus elevate—her candidacy.

Message to the hiring manager:
I am excited to complete my Clinical Fellowship Year (CFY) in a challenging hospital/rehabilitation setting. I possesses a great deal of energy and enthusiasm for working with individuals with neurogenic communicate disorders. I believe I could make a very positive contribution to your rehabilitative team!

Resume:

EDUCATION

Master of Science in Communicative Disorders (May 1996)
Major in Speech-Language Pathology
University of Wisconsin-Madison

Bachelor of Arts in Communicative Disorders (May 1994)
University of Wisconsin-Madison
Dean's List (1990–1994)
Member, Golden Key National Honor Society (1991–present)

CERTIFICATION   CCC-SLP (pending completion of CFY)

SPECIAL SKILLS

— Certified in Porch Index of Communicate Ability (PICA) administration
— Augmentative and Alternative communication system programming familiarity
— Systematic Analysis of Language Transcripts (SALT) experience
— Basic Signed English skills
— Word processing familiarity (Microsoft Word, WordPerfect)
— Computer literate, particularly with Macintosh systems

CLINICAL EXPERIENCE

Student Clinician

MONROE HOSPITAL (Spring 1996)
— Provided speech/language/cognitive/swallowing assessment and treatment for adults and children
— Participated in home care rehabilitation
— Provided speech/language/cognitive intervention for adults with developmental disabilities

GRIEF COUNSELOR

TEACHER—GRIEF AND BEREAVEMENT COUNSELING

EMPLOYMENT DESIRED:
Mid-Atlantic region desired (VA, MD, DC, NC).
– Teaching at post-secondary or graduate level biological sciences or allied health
– Grief and bereavement counseling
– Funeral Service Profession—teaching or management

PROFESSIONAL EXPERTISE / SKILLS:
Specialized Managerial Training: Coping with Disruptive Students - Interactive Computer Technologies - Fundamentals of Human Resources - Sexual Harassment - Assessment and Evaluation - Total Quality Management/TQM - Conflict Management in the Workplace - PA Act 148 / AIDS Confidentiality - Accreditation Site-Team Evaluation.

Specialized Funeral Service Training: Advanced Embalming, Cosmetology and Restorative Art Techniques - Grief, Bereavement, Perinatal Loss and Suicide Counseling - Funeral Home Management and Software Applications - OSHA Standards and Respiratory Protection - Handling of Infectious, Contagious, and Communicable Disease Cases - Preceptor's Training for Funeral Directors.

WORK HISTORY:
Director/Assistant Professor, Department of Funeral Service Education, Northhampton Community College, Bethlehem, PA
1988–present.
– Development and maintenance of program
– Teaching of general pathology, embalming, and restorative art courses
– Staff development and assessment
– Student counseling, advising, recruitment, and retention
– Computer software applications, multimedia presentations
Licensed Funeral Director/Embalmer, Commonwealth of PA, 1988–present.
Assistant Manager, Colonial Funeral Home, Falls Church, VA 1987–1988
– Director of embalming operations
– Development of in-house computer operations
Funeral Service Licensee, Commonwealth of VA 1985–present.
Funeral Service Trainee/Licensee, Money and King Vienna Funeral Home, Vienna, VA 1983–86
– Assistant director of embalming
– Accounts receivable collection

EDUCATIONAL BACKGROUND:
– Certified Perinatal Loss Counselor, Penn State Univ./Milton S. Hershey Medical Center, Hershey, PA, 1995.
– M.Ed. Education Administration, Lehigh Univ., Bethlehem, PA, 1992.
– Certified Funeral Service Practitioner, Academy of Professional Funeral Service Practice, Lanham, MD, 1991.
– BS Mortuary Science, Xavier Univ., Cincinnati, OH, 1983.
– Certified Eye Enucleation and Homograph Eardrum Autopsy Retrieval/HEAR Technician, Cincinnati College of Mortuary Science, Cincinnati, OH, 1983.
– AAS Mortuary Science, Cincinnati College of Mortuary Science, Cincinnati, OH 1983.

SPECIAL AWARDS/ACCOMPLISHMENTS:
Published Works
– Summative Personality Trait Evaluation
– Futures Perspective for Funeral Service Education
– Infectious Waste Control College-Wide Plan
– Self-Study Report to the Committee on Accreditation/American Board of Funeral Service
– Academic Audit and Annual Report: Department of Funeral Service Practice
– Contributing Author—Embalming: History, Theory, and Practice
– OSHA Standards Compliance Manual for Funeral Directors

PROFESSIONAL ORGANIZATIONS:
- Board of Trustees, Academy of Professional Funeral Practice—1993–present.
- Secretary/Treasurer, Academy of Professional Funeral Service Practice—1994–present.
- Chairperson, Education and Disaster Preparedness Committees, Eastern Pennsylvania Funeral Directors Association—1994–present.
- Member, Finance Committee, American Board of Funeral Service Education—1991–present.

SPECIAL INTERESTS:
Family Activities - Outdoor Activities - Helping others through teaching - Computer applications

PERSONAL/PROFESSIONAL REFERENCES:
Available Upon Request.

Transmitted: 95-08-18 11:41:47 EDT

A relatively effective résumé, but the three distinct Objectives (under "Employment Desired") make the candidate appear unfocused. He'd be better off saving his teaching ambitions for a separate résumé, marketed specifically to secondary school and technical college situations. He can then more effectively tailor each résumé to a distinct opportunity.

CHAPTER 20

Marketing Yourself Effectively

There are a number of ways to get the word out that you exist and are available. In this chapter, you will learn how to catalog and set priorities for those methods that work best for you.

Marketing yourself successfully requires more than simply answering want ads, contacting recruiters, and throwing your résumé on the Internet. You need an edge. Often it's you against a vast number of other men and women who also want the job as badly as you do. Both timing and approach can be critical. But there are unconventional methods that can be even more effective, which allow you to be the first to apply for a job, or, in some instances, to create your own job. So on the theory that the arsenal with the most weapons is the best one, here is a list of the conventional and unconventional sources you can use to find a job:

- Employment agencies
- Executive search firms
- Newspaper want ads and business section display ads
- Industry or function journals and newsletters
- Industry association officers and members
- Former coworkers and other professional networks
- The Internet, quickly becoming one of the most effective sources of all

Here are the merits of each of these job sources:

EMPLOYMENT AGENCIES

Find out which agencies in your metropolitan area are active in healthcare in general and your function in particular, then call a counselor at each of them. Only after you have the name of a live human being who specializes in your field should you send a résumé and cover letter. That way you will have a personal emissary in each office who can be on the lookout for opportunities that may interest you. Be prepared to rework your résumé if the counselor feels this will improve your chances.

Employment agencies work primarily in the interests of client employers because that's where they make their money. So do not expect to find agents who will work exclusively for you. They will help you if they think you can help them earn a fee. This is not because employment agents are callous people, but because in their business they simply do not have the time to both counsel and make a living. You will get numerous good tips from most of them when you ask specific questions. Just don't expect them to spend a lot of time actively protecting your interests.

Be sure to arrange at least one personal interview at each agency. Try to present yourself as an individual, not just a résumé. This definitely will improve your chances.

Call your counselor every other week or so—not so often that you become a nuisance, but often enough to be kept in mind. Chances are far less than 50–50 that you'll find your next job through an employment agency. Still, it is only common sense to spread your name around as widely as possible. Each call will take just 60 to 90 seconds out of your day, and you may just remind an unorganized counselor that there is indeed an opening for which you should be considered.

EXECUTIVE RECRUITERS

The big difference between employment agencies and recruiters is that the headhunters tend to work with higher-salaried people. There are two types of executive recruiters: retainer firms (which get their money up front, regardless of whether they get the job done or not), and contingency firms (which don't get paid until a placement is made). Retainer firms tend to look down on contingency firms, but the quality of work done by both is essentially the same.

Treat your relationship with any recruiter the way you would an employment agency counselor, with the understanding that their allegiance is to the client company rather than to you.

Become Your Own Trend Spotter

If you want to spot new business opportunities before anyone else, says Robert Tucker, president of The Innovative Resource in Sherman Oaks, California, you have to have a well-thought-out strategy for gathering information on what's going on around you. Tucker outlines seven steps to becoming a successful trend spotter:

1) *Audit your information intake.* Do the publications you read or the colleagues you associate with provide you with information you can really put to use?
2) *Develop front-line observational skills.* Draw your own conclusions about what's happening in the world. Do not rely just on newspaper or television accounts.

3) *Ask questions.* Take a journalism course in basic interviewing. You can learn a lot more from people if you know how to ask questions and listen actively.

4) *Do as professional trend watchers do.* Here's a lesson from author John Naisbitt: Reading small-town newspapers can clue you into significant changes that start at the grassroots level.

5) *Make your reading time count.* Skip over gossip or disaster stories and concentrate on articles that contain thoughtful analyses. Look for what's different, incongruous, worrisome, exciting.

6) *Organize your information.* Silicon Valley marketing consultant Regis McKenna reads between 50 and 100 magazines a week. He clips articles and creates files for information he wants to keep.

7) *Monitor all information-rich media.* Turn off the TV and listen to a radio call-in show or a recorded "publication" like the Hines Report, a monthly audiocassette service that updates events in the business and financial community.

Here is a wrinkle you might try to exploit. Recruiters sometimes try to generate business by introducing outstanding candidates to a prospective client just to demonstrate the caliber of candidates they work with. To elevate your candidacy to this level, inform your counselor (if he or she works this way) of your strengths, particularly as they relate to the local marketplace. Find out what openings the firm is working on and what specific fields your counselor handles successfully. If you can sell yourself enough to convince an agent to make a few cold calls on your behalf, you will be that much further ahead.

To check out recruiters who are likely to have something at your level and in your specialty, write or call the American Management Association (AMA), 1601 Broadway, New York, NY 10036; (212) 586-8100; FAX (212) 903-8163 for a copy of its *Executive Employment Guide.* For $20, you will receive a list of more than 125 executive recruiters nationwide (several with offices world-wide), including names; phone numbers; special fields covered, if any; minimum salaries of positions handled; and an indication of whether each accepts résumés or will accede to an interview about opportunities in general. The entries are cross-referenced both by city and state and by job specialty. Another source is *The Directory of Executive Recruiters,* from Kennedy Publications (Templeton Road, Fitzwilliam, NH 03447); (800) 531-0138; FAX (603) 585-9555). At $39.95, it's twice the price of the AMA guide, but it does list more than 2,800 search firms in the United States, Canada, and Mexico, and the entries are as inclusive as those in the AMA guide. If you have access to a well stocked public library, you may be able to avoid buying either book.

NEWSPAPER WANT ADS AND HEALTHCARE SECTION DISPLAY ADS

Responding to newspaper ads can be a frustrating experience, because there is often no feedback after you've taken the time and effort to put together a tailored résumé and letter. Still, there is always the possibility that an ad will lead to your next position. So once you accept it for the long shot it is, you can devote as much time responding to ads as they deserve.

A good way to keep your ad-answering campaign in perspective is to rate all of the ads you consider as 1s, 2s, or 3s, against the following criteria:

It's a 1 if: The ad reads like a mirror of your résumé.

Strategy: Act as though you personally had been asked to be considered for the position. Research the hiring organization extensively so that you can demonstrate in your cover letter a knowledge of the employer that you couldn't get from reading the ad alone. (See research sources at the beginning of Chapter 21.) Edit your résumé objective or summary to the extent that each includes all aspects of your background that match the employer's needs. Write a cover letter that answers the ad's requirements point for point, in the same sequence they were written. Write—and then rewrite—a description of those accomplishments, skills, and responsibilities that relate specifically to each requirement, and delete all excess words.

Tactic: Wait a least a week before sending off your ad response. Most applicants think that the first résumés received make the strongest impression. But what usually happens is that the earliest to arrive just get lost in an avalanche of letters and résumés. Many "first readers" actually spend less time on each of the first several hundred responses to arrive than they do on those arriving a week later.

It's a 2 if: The job is a near match. You can easily satisfy four of the five or six requirements specified for the position. In short, you know you can do the job.

Strategy: Give the letter at least an hour of your time, checking off those of your accomplishments and skills that match up with the stated requirement. Stress your advertisement-related strengths to make up for the one or two credentials you may lack.

Tactic: As you would for a **1**, wait a week before responding, and try to learn something about the institution.

It's a 3 if: The job sounds good. It may be a stretch for you the way it is described, but you think you could handle it.

Strategy: Give it a "short-term best shot"—your résumé accompanied by a letter stating your qualifications as powerfully as you can. But don't spend a lot of time on it; there are probably a large number of applicants ahead of you.

Tactic: Again, wait before you send it off.

There is also a fourth rating for newspaper ads worth mentioning. Often an ad will suggest additional jobs after the first position is filled. A new chief of anatomic pathology, for example, may need one or more pathologist assistants after settling into the job. If a number-two slot suggests itself and you believe you could fill it, put the ad in a "suspense" file, for further reference. Call periodically to see if the job has been filled, and ask for an interview when you get through to the right person. The downside: Filling the first job may take several months before candidates are considered for jobs generated by it.

Blind Ads

Some ads that do not identify the advertiser will be extremely appealing and seem to have only you in mind. The rub is that no matter how attractive the ad, there is little chance that you will get a response. Here's why:

Institutions that do not identify themselves need not worry about any bad publicity generated by not responding to application letters; therefore, you never hear from them unless they are sure you are an exact fit. Other blind ads are placed by executive recruiters hired to find a candidate for a specific job. Your chances of getting an interview rest entirely on whether you are perceived by the recruiter as a viable candidate. Your chances of hearing from the recruiter, then, are close to nil.

Other blind ads are placed by employers who have decided to replace one or more of their employees, but are reluctant to take action until they find a suitable replacement. They don't want word to get out that there is a problem and thereby damage employee morale—not to mention the aid and comfort it would provide the competition.

TRADE PUBLICATION ARTICLES AND CLASSIFIED ADS

Spend a half day every week at the best medical, public, or college library available, and assemble an intelligence system effective enough to anticipate trends that may in turn trigger job openings. Go through trade magazines in your area of specialty or interest, such as *American Journal of Clinical Nutrition, The American Nurse, Hospital and Health Services Administration, and Radiologic Journal.* This is a good way to keep up with specialty trends. Identify contact people or possible employers, and scan any classifieds for openings of interest to you. A good source directory for healthcare trade magazines is *Magazine Industry Marketplace,* revised annually and available at most libraries.

DATABASE SERVICES

Most public libraries also use one or more of a number of database services offered by a growing number of providers. Here are five of the most popular:
- Infotrac: A journal and newspaper article index providing data about prospective employers
- Business Dateline OnDisc: Business articles appearing in local, state, and regional journals, newspapers, and magazines, that are of interest to job seekers
- ProQuest: Business articles in newspapers and magazines
- Standard & Poor's Corporation: Listings of public and private companies as well as biographical listings
- Ultimate Job Finder: 4,500 sources of trade and specialty journals

INDUSTRY AND FUNCTION ASSOCIATION OFFICERS AND MEMBERS

Membership directories are great sources for identifying leaders in your field who are also potential contacts. Consult *Directories in Print* (Volumes I and II), updated annually, and look up your targeted association from the directory in the appropriate, alphabetically listed specialty.

FORMER COWORKERS AND OTHER PROFESSIONAL NETWORKS

To identify employers that have or may soon have openings, contact former colleagues or friends in other hospitals, clinics, or institutions to see who knows somebody in power at each target employer, and arrange an information interview. In its most professional form, this systematic method of contacting and follow-up is called networking. It is one way to find out before you read it in the classifieds that a job is about to open up. An overwhelming majority of positions do not get advertised because they are filled quickly by people who have done their homework and have tapped into the networks mentioned in this chapter. This is what you may have heard referred to as the "hidden job market." There is no need to advertise, after all, if qualified candidates for a position have already been found.

The trick is for you to become one of those candidates. You can do that by identifying a hospital or clinic you would like to work for, and then finding one or more inside contacts to provide you with information. To help you determine whether an opening exists or might soon exist, ask as many of the following questions as you can, and any others you can think of:

- Is there an impending merger or acquisition?
- Is expansion likely—or the addition of one or more services?
- Is profitability up—and likely to remain there?
- Are any new activities scheduled that may require someone with your capabilities?
- Is the employer experiencing any particular problems that a person with your background could help solve?

Here is a series of questions to ask yourself that will help you set up your own network, and help you test the cliché, "It's not what you know, it's who you know":

Who do you know who is employed by an institution you might want to work for?

....
....
....

Who do you know who does the kind of work you want to be hired to do?

....
....
....

Who do you know who seems to be well connected?

....
....
....

Who do you know (even if only slightly) from professional or trade associations?

....
....
....

Who do you know from your last job who would be willing to put you in touch with others?

....
....
....

Who else did you come into contact with in your last job who might have leads (e.g., suppliers, customers, patients)?

....
....
....

Who do you know from school, rotations, or alumni associations who might have contacts or be good for contacts themselves?

....
....
....

Who in your extended family might be able to help?

....
....
....

The idea in networking is to get those you contact initially to refer you to others. Whether you come up with five names or fifty, the number of your contacts will grow as you ask each person you approach for the names of two or three others you might talk to.

Locum Tenens: Physicians as Temps

Locum tenens is the Latin term for someone holding a place. In the medical profession it refers to physicians who hold temporary positions for other physicians who must be absent from their practices. Locum tenens physicians fill vacancies in solo practices, on hospital staffs, and in managed care organizations. Assignments can range from one week to a year. Today there is a growing demand for locum tenens physicians, especially during times of peak patient load, such as flu season. Practices can more easily balance staffing shortages without burdening the permanent staff.

A contact interview, whether in person or on the phone, should be viewed as an opportunity to promote your job-worthiness.

Most people are flattered when asked their advice, and will be particularly willing to help if you are a friend of a friend (or, even better, a relative of a friend)—as long as you respect their time and are prepared to ask informed questions. If you are new to your target specialty, this will involve research. Do not ask your contacts to investigate job opportunities for you. You put them in an awkward position, and a subsequent call will likely go unreturned.

To maximize the value of your network, always get at least one additional name during the course of any phone or in-person interview. Record your networking contacts in a notebook for easy access and follow-up. Here are column headings for vital information that will allow you to do this (the "Source" column will allow you to keep track of individuals who provided names of people you have contacted):

NAME	COMPANY	TITLE	ADDRESS	PHONE	RESULTS	SOURCE	FOLLOW-UP

NETWORKING ONLINE

If you are a stranger to online and Internet sources as part of your job-search strategy, you are missing more than you realize. One way to rectify this is to visit your local book store. Spend some time leafing through specific books before making an investment. Two to consider are *The Complete Idiot's Guide to the Internet* (Peter Kent, Macmillan, $19.95) and *The Internet Guide for New Users* (Daniel Dern, McGraw-Hill, $27.95).

If you have a computer and have not yet selected a commercial online service, here are five worth considering. Because this is such an emerging and highly competitive industry, the list may look very different six months after this book is published. Prices and available benefits vary widely from service to service, often from one month to the next. Most of the five services listed below offer a trial membership, so your initial decision need not be a costly one; try at least two for comparison purposes.

America Online
8619 Westwood Center Drive
Vienna, VA 22182
(800) 848-8199
FAX (703) 883-1509

GEnie
401 N. Washington Street
Rockville, MD 20850
(800) 638-9636

CompuServe
5000 Arlington Centre Boulevard
Columbus, OH 43220
(800) 848-8199
FAX (614) 457-0348

Prodigy
445 Hamilton Avenue
White Plains, NY 10601
(800) 776-3449

Delphi Internet
1030 Massachusetts Avenue
Cambridge, MA 02138
(800) 695-4005
FAX (617) 491-6642

All five of these commercial services offer networking opportunities and job-search capabilities in the healthcare industry. Through their interactive special interest areas (called "forums," "bulletin boards," or "newsgroups," depending on the service), you can often zero in on your own specialty, introduce yourself, state your need, offer whatever kind of reciprocal assistance you can to other users, and wait for the responses to come in. CompuServe, for example, offers several options. Let's walk through one:

1) *From the services listed on the CompuServe Information Service screen, click "Professional." (This activates your modem to get you online.)*
2) *From the list that appears, click "Health/Medical."*
3) *In that list you have 16 options, eight of which cover medical specialties. To keep the demonstration simple, click the first item, "AMIA Medical Forum." (Other possibilities include "Public Health Forum," "Business Database Plus," "Physicians Data Query," and "Comprehensive Core Medical Library," all of which offer networking assistance.)*
4) *Once in "MedSIG," you will have a number of ways to access assistance. For now, click "browse messages."*
5) *From that menu of 21 topics (which change periodically), click "Students and Employment." (Other possibilities today include "Dental"—69 topics, 336 messages; "Nursing"—31 topics, 85 messages; and "Mental Health"—52 topics, 558 messages.)*

6) Under "Students/Employment" are 16 messages under the subtopic "Pursuing a Career in Medicine." One high school senior wants to know what coursework he should be taking. "I plan on talking to the college counselor, but I'd like to get some info beforehand . . . ." Three doctors have replied with on-target advice. (Perhaps some of it would apply to your situation.) You can read strangers' mail here! And not only does nobody care, they want you to jump in, too. Another writer asks if there is an age limit on starting medical school. Among the several responses: "It may not be your chronological age that is the largest factor, but your lifetime goals and how they fit with your career goals." This networking effort was the result of following a single "thread" in one small part of a part of a single online service. And the options are virtually limitless. (Among the alternatives in the "Students/Employment" listing in the CompuServe MedSIG forum, for example, was "Career Match Database," "Nevada M.D. Wanted," "International Employment," and a recently graduated student seeking "Medical Assisting.") See the following list of MedSIG message sections available.

The other commercial services offer similar networking opportunities. A Health Professionals Network, as well as a Nurses Network, is available from America Online. Delphi also has a Nursing Network forum. Prodigy includes veterinary, medical, and nursing forums. Ask for a demonstration before you sign up with any of them, and go with the service that offers more of what you want than the others.

MedSIG Message Sections: A Sampling

(Annotations are by CompuServe)

1. General/Professional
   General news and comments about health professions
2. Office Systems
   Material relating to medical computer office systems
3. Clinical/Consulting
   Clinical questions and clinical consulting
4. Students and Employment
   Medical/nursing students and other health professional students; employment opportunities in healthcare delivery or management
5. FP/Peds/OB-GYN
   Family practice, pediatrics, and OB/GYN topics
6. Subspecialties
   Nonprimary care specialists and their concerns and issues
7. CCM/ED/Pre-Hosp
   Critical care, emergency department, and paramedic/EMT message section
8. Nursing
   Nursing informatics and professional issues

9. Journal Club/CME

    Monthly *Journal of American Medical Association* club threads and other CME activities

10. Research/Bioethics

    Discussions about medical science, bioethics, biostatistics

11. Informatics

    Discussions of medical informatics, artificial intelligence/neural nets, medical computing and systems development, as well as Internet and telemedicine issues

12. Health Policy/Legal

    Managed care, health reform, as well as other legal and health policy issues

13. Dental

    Dental informatics, treatment, prevention, networking

14. TQM/QI/Med Record

    The Quality Movement in Medicine interface; electronic medical record, medical management science and related topics

15. PA/Allied Health

    This section is for the discussion of physician assistant and allied health professions issues and concerns

16. Mental Health

    All facets of mental health and illness

17. The Lounge

    Everyone gets an honorary Ph.D. while visiting MedSIG, so relax and enjoy yourself

18. Marketplace

    Discussions by vendors of their products, low-level general customer support questions, wanted to buy or for-sale items of medical or computer equipment

19. Pharm/Rx

    Message section for pharmacists and pharmacy discussions, as well as questions about drugs, drug use, and medical treatments

20. Lab/Dx

    Laboratory medicine and pathology discussions. Low-level customer support for laboratory information systems. Discussions of other diagnostic modalities, such as medical imaging

21. Palmtops/Laptops

    Laptops, notebooks, subnotebooks, palmtops, personal digital assistants, paging systems/cellular communications hardware and software discussions

22. International

    MedSIG has participation from around the world. Because of the numbers involved, much of the emphasis has been on the United States and Canada. This section is currently under construction.

Job Search on the Internet

For more formal job search, extra effort is involved getting on the Internet, as well as its access system, the World Wide Web. For those of you not yet there, you need a computer that can handle graphics, and a fast modem. Your computer processor should be at least a 486, the modem no slower than 14,400K baud, and preferably 28,800K. You will also need Internet browsing software, which varies depending on the online service you use (one of the commercial services introduced on page 264, or a "regional provider"). A knowledgeable customer service rep at the nearest large computer store will help you out. Also read *Free Stuff From the Internet* by Patrick Vincent (Coriolis Group Books, 1995) for a chapter on mastering the intricacies of Internet job search, and *Hook Up, Get Hired!*, by Joyce Lain Kennedy (Wiley, 1995), an entire book devoted to job-searching on the Internet—including several healthcare industry sources. As for specific organizations maintaining web sites, here are several:

The Centers for Disease Control maintains a World Wide Web homepage covering healthcare employment opportunities, including current job openings, student employment opportunities, general employment opportunities, and education and training opportunities. (You can also reach this source by mail at 1600 Clifton Rd. NE, Atlanta, GA 30333.)

Cool Career Sites is the most comprehensive center for job-search services we are aware of. Here is what is available through its various links:

- MedSearch America: Specializing in healthcare-related jobs. Capabilities include searching for jobs, posting your résumé (sample MedSearch résumés can be found on pages 232–255), viewing profiles of featured employers, and posting your own ad of unlimited length for up to two months. Open to any individual, group, company, or organization from the healthcare community. Membership is free for job seekers at http://www.medsearch.com or call (206) 883-7252 for additional information.
- Career Magazine: Search the job listings, or add your résumé to the online Résumé Bank (http:www.jobline.com/jobline).
- CareerMosaic: Resources for new college graduates
- CareerNet: An array of career resources and links to thousands of sites
- CareerSite: Thousands of free listings, in addition to "Virtual Agent" services
- CareerWEB: Global recruitment and resource center
- Chicago Tribune's Career Finder: Job opportunities, company profiles, articles, and more
- E-Span: Up-to-date resources for job-seekers and employers
- Helpwanted.com: Jobs listed by company
- IntelliMatch: A service that matches online résumés with job skill profiles
- JobWeb: Career planning, employment information, articles, tips, and more
- The Monster Board: Résumés, job postings, and employer profiles
- NationJob Network: Searchable database of postings from across the United States, primarily the Midwest

- Online Career Center: A nonprofit association of employers offering the Internet's most frequently accessed career center
- PeopleBank: International listings for employers and job-seekers alike
- Virtual Job Fair: Research and scan through potential employers

Best of all, every "cool career site" is accessible through a single World Wide Web address: http://www.infoseek.com/doc/netdir/career.html

CHAPTER 21

Winning Interview Techniques

The key to generating interviews that lead to job offers is preparation. The more knowledgeable you are about your prospective employers, the easier it will be for them to visualize you on their payroll. But first, they must be able to see how you can help them solve their problems, provide better care, or save them money.[1]

KNOW YOUR PROSPECTIVE EMPLOYERS

Make it your business to learn as much as you can about the employer before the interview, including the job you are interviewing for and your prospective boss. You can go about this in several ways, depending on how you found out about the position in the first place: through an advertisement, from a recruiter or agency, or by networking, either on or off the Internet.

Advertisements in Newspapers, Trade Journals, or Newsletters

If a company identifies itself, there are several ways you can gather data about it. For instance, publicly held companies are required by the Securities and Exchange Commission to report various kinds of information, all of which are available to the public in a number of business directories. Some of these directories specialize by industry, others by size. In general, more information is available for the larger, publicly held companies, although Dun & Bradstreet's *Million Dollar Directory* lists the top 50,000 companies with a net worth of more than $500,000. Increasing numbers of companies provide information on the Internet, as well, through home pages in several business-oriented databases.

---

[1] For medical students preparing for residency selection, *Strolling Through the Match* (American Academy of Family Physicians) is an excellent handbook covering curriculum vitae writing, choosing a specialty, interviewing tips, and follow-up.

General Interest Reference Books and Industry-Specific Directories

Business Organizations, Agencies, and Publications Directory

Corporate 1000

Directory of Corporate Affiliations

Directories in Print (Volumes I and II)

Dun's Million Dollar Directory (Volumes I, II, and III)

Encyclopedia of Business Information Sources

International Corporate 1000

Macmillan Directory of Leading Private Companies

Small Business Sourcebook

Standard Directory of Advertisers

Probably the most informative of these directories is the *Directory of Corporate Affiliations,* which is published annually and updated with bimonthly supplements. An index in an accompanying volume lists more than 40,000 divisions, subsidiaries, affiliates, and parent companies, and the page on which the complete listing of each appears. This is followed by extensive genealogies for the more than 4,000 parent companies, including address, telephone number, stock exchange or exchanges, approximate annual sales, number of employees, type of business, and top corporate officers. It also lists all divisions, subsidiaries, affiliates, and so on, with address, telephone number, type of business, and name of chief operating officer.

Additional geographical and Standard Industrial Code (S.I.C.) indexes list all companies by city and state, and primary types of business, respectively. The *Directory of Corporate Affiliations* is one of the few commercial reference works that effectively keeps up with the growing whirlwind of acquisitions and mergers. Your interest probably will lie in S.I.C.s 8000–8999, which cover larger doctor's offices, hospitals, clinics, laboratories, and nursing care facilities.

Other general interest and industry-specific directories listed above should help you as well. If you do not see your specialty, ask your local or medical librarian for suggestions. You might start with *Directories in Print,* published semi-annually, which is exactly what it says it is. Remember, though, that no matter where you get your information, it is to your advantage to go into an interview knowing the full range of an employer's products and services, including recent projections of long-term strategies and objectives. Also, check out the special issues of leading business and healthcare magazines as a source for annually updated information.

Another good way to gather information about for-profit target employers is to call for their most recent annual reports, as well as any descriptive literature that might be illuminating. An annual report will give you a better handle on a company's financial status and its growth strategy, and perhaps confirm clues to its "culture." Call the public information department, specifically its department of investor relations, if it is publicly held. (In answer to what probably will be the first question, say yes: You might indeed become a stockholder if a few things go the right way.)

Many not-for-profit institutions—larger hospitals, for example—publish annual reports as well, usually for employees rather than stockholders. They include much valuable information, but often skimp on the financial information. See what more a polite call to the public relations department will produce.

Other sources of information are former colleagues (or neighbors, family members, or friends) who may know somebody at an executive level. Under the best of circumstances you may be able to learn the name of the person hiring for the position, and something about his or her background and management style. You may also get additional information about the company, perhaps including reasons why the position is open and who held it most recently. If you can get to the person who left the job, you may pick up valuable information (but perhaps misinformation as well, especially if the person left under duress).

Finally, go back over the ad that got you the interview in the first place. Memorize every nuance of every requirement. Your answers should all be framed by what you know the employer is looking for. Here's an exercise to help you prepare[2]:

PREPARING FOR YOUR INTERVIEW

Whether your interview was set up by a search firm or an employment agency, or was the result of your answering an ad, the first part of your preparation should be focused on the company itself. Answer as many questions as you can from the list below.

What position does the employer want to fill?
....
....
....

What attracted you to the job?
....
....
....

Reading between the lines, what do you think the company is really looking for?
....
....
....

---
[2] Exercises in this chapter are based on JOB-BRIDGE, a career transition program © Wilson McLeran, Inc., New Haven, CT 06511.

What are the skills needed for the job? (e.g., initiative, working well under pressure, problem solving, expertise with any special medical equipment)
....
....
....

For each of the skills you have identified, list specific examples of instances in which you have demonstrated that skill. (Space is provided for four skills.)
1. ....
....
....
2. ....
....
....
3. ....
....
....
4. ....
....
....

Investigating the Position Through an Agency Source

If you are working with an executive recruiter or employment agency counselor who is an effective professional, you have little to worry about. Because they live by the client fees generated by the people they place, recruiters certainly are not going to relax if they sense that you may be one of their next placements. They will coach you to say everything they think will benefit you in the interview. Nevertheless, some recruiters are a lot more efficient than others. And it is those "others" who can ruin your efforts if you do not take an assertive posture.

Here are some vital facts and figures you will need to help you prepare for the interview. If your recruiter or agency counselor has not already supplied it, ask for information in the following categories:

1) *Employer (adapt for type of institution)*
   - *Patient volume (this year; last two years)*
   - *Nurse:patient ratio (this year; last two years)*
   - *Number of employees*
   - *Growth prospects; strengths and weaknesses*
   - *Patient care philosophy*
   - *Possible problems; why they exist; how they might be overcome*

2) *Position*
   - *Why is it open? (When was it last open, and why?)*
   - *How long has it been open? (If two months or more: Why so tough to fill?)*
   - *Where is the person who previously held it? (Can we talk to him/her?)*
   - *How many people have been interviewed so far?*
   - *How many candidates are still in the running? (Why are they still being considered?)*
   - *What are the prospects for advancement?*
   - *What do you think will be the determining factor in getting the job?*
   - *Why do you think I am still a candidate?*
   - *How many others are doing the same work?*
   - *What is the salary policy? How are raises determined? How good is the benefits program?*
   - *How will performance be measured?*
3) *Boss*
   - *Title?*
   - *Background? Previous experience?*
   - *How long with the employer?*
   - *Do you know him/her personally, or have you talked only with human resources?*
   - *What are his or her prospects with the company?*

VARIOUS NETWORKING AND RESEARCH LEADS

If you have researched a company that interests you and written a good enough letter to be rewarded with an interview, call the person you heard from and ask what the specific focus of your meeting will be, so you can prepare. Also ask if there is any company literature or material that could be sent to you. Keep in mind, though, that because of where you have worked or what you have accomplished, the interviewer may simply want to pick your brain and may not have a job in mind at all.

This is your calculated risk: sometimes interviews such as this are a waste of time. Never mind. You can often turn such a situation to your advantage.

The name of this game is "marketplace." Let's assume that you do have information of value to your interviewer about your current company or its competitors, or about some of the people at one or more of these companies. First determine that this interview will not likely lead to a job offer. Answer the first couple of questions put to you—within bounds of industry ethics, of course. (For example, you should reveal no proprietary information about, say, growth plans or policy decisions that have not yet been made public.) Then ask a couple of questions of your own, even if it means changing the subject. You need to address *your* agenda relatively early in the conversation while you still have an advantage.

Examples:

"What's happening over at MDS labs with that biomedical management program they said was such a breakthrough?"

"Who's looking for a good ultrasonographer?"

"I've heard there's some activity at (interviewer's previous employer, institution whose top management is known to interviewer). Is it OK if I use your name in trying to set up an interview there?"

"(Name of subsidiary of interviewer's company or other company known well by interviewer) interests me considerably. Who should I talk with there to introduce myself? What do you think they are looking for?"

Remember, you will do the best job at the interview by coming in extremely well prepared. And if you have information of your own that might be of value, now is the time to get as much data as you can in return.

THE FIRST INTERVIEW

To dispose of the worst news first: The job does not always go to the most qualified. Even though most human resource interviewers are skilled at their jobs and pass along to the line executives those candidates who seem to fulfill the requirements for an open position, the direct supervisor often lacks good interviewing skills. On what basis, then, are many hiring decisions made? First impressions.

First Impressions

Given two or more candidates with similar credentials, the job will almost invariably go to the person who projects honesty, sincerity, and enthusiasm. Those of you who are nurses or who spend much of your on-duty time in direct patient or public contact will be judged on the empathy and compassion you project, as well. Your physical appearance, mannerisms, vocabulary, attitude, and nonverbal communication all contribute to the impression you make.

Your feeling of confidence can singularly affect a first impression. That confidence, in turn, can be generated initially by something as fundamental as sound preparation. Don't underestimate it. It becomes a self-fulfilling prophecy. Your confidence level will lead to an attitude that the employer needs you, rather than the other way around. *Feel* successful and chances are better that you will be successful.

Before the interview, go over the résumé you have provided the interviewer beforehand. (If you have written more than one version, be sure to have the differences straight in your head.) Treat every résumé entry as if it were a script cue. You were brought in for an interview initially because your professional credentials were of interest. If you have been able to find out what triggered the specific interest in you, that puts you ahead of the game. One way to determine this is to go over your résumé line by line to anticipate which of your qualities have generated the employer's interest in you. Think of responses to questions that will allow you to elaborate on your accomplishments. For example, the interviewer may ask:

"You say here that as a lab technician you assess body composition using a dual-energy C-ray absorptionmeter. Would you mind taking me through that process, step by step?"

This kind of follow-up question gives you the opportunity to go into enough detail that will assure your prospective boss:

—that you are fully capable of handling this aspect of the job (they ask because it is important to them) and

—that your résumé is both accurate and balanced.

First interviews should be viewed as one-shot opportunities. As such, rehearse all résumé-entry elaborations as though this were the only chance you have to tell your story, because that may well be the case. Be able to talk lucidly from ten seconds to ten minutes about any given résumé entry, depending on where the interviewer's interest lies.

Here is a good way to get this done to your satisfaction, as well as the interviewer's.

Preparing to Answer Résumé Questions

Keeping in mind the requirements for the job and what you believe the employer is looking for, use your résumé to prepare discussing your accomplishments. In the left-hand column, list all accomplishments mentioned on your résumé. In the right-hand column, explain why and how you attained them.

Accomplishment	Why and how Attained
1.	....
....	....
....	....
2.	....
....	....
....	....
3.	....
....	....
....	....
4.	....
....	....
....	....
5.	....
....	....
....	....
6.	....
....	....
....	....
7.	....
....	....
....	....

Responding to Tough Questions

Though every interview is different, all will include one or more questions that you would just as soon not have to answer. The interviewer will be listening not only for content but also for sincerity, poise, and an ability to think quickly. Spend some time before you interview developing answers to questions you think might give you trouble. Some of them may be tough and fair. Some of them may be tough and unfair.

Everyone has an "obnoxious question threshold" past which he or she cannot, or should not, go. A question you consider beyond fairness calls for an appropriate response. For example, if you feel it is an invasion of your privacy to take an employer-administered polygraph test, say so. Never compromise strongly held personal beliefs or values to score interview points. If you have heard enough to tell you that this institution's values differ markedly from your own, terminate the interview politely on these appropriate grounds. After all, if you and the employer are far apart philosophically before you are hired, it can only get worse after you come on board.

If you recently left a job, the reason will undoubtedly come up at the interview. Answer this question truthfully and briefly. If you were fired because your performance or attitude was in question, indicate the extent to which you have made this a learning experience, and the extent to which you have profited from it. Try to anticipate additional questions intended to get more details about your termination, and rehearse your answers repeatedly.

This is a key stage of the interview. If you can get beyond this early mine field, you will be able to concentrate on more positive and productive matters.

Most interviewers ask one or more tough questions. Some interviewers seem to ask nothing but tough questions. Basically, they simply want to know what you can offer the institution and fairly catalog your strengths and weaknesses. After writing answers to the questions that follow, memorize and rehearse them.

What do you know about us? (Do the research so you will have some key information.)
....
....
....

Why do you want to work for us? (Words and phrases to think about in formulating your answer: challenge, industry leader, quality of healthcare, growth potential.)
....
....
....

What would you do for us? What can you do for us that someone else can't? (Relate your answer in terms of the employer's needs.)
....
....
....

What about this position do you find the most attractive? the least attractive? (Careful! Think in terms of long-term professional growth.)
....
....
....

Why should we hire you? (Not because you need a job. Think about specific contributions you can make.)
....
....
....

You appear to be overqualified for the position we have to offer. Do you agree? (This comment often speaks to your age, or sometimes your salary level. Think of ways your experience could be an asset, and address a possible employer objection related to fitting in with younger team members or a younger boss. Present yourself as up-to-date and current. This is no time to reminisce about your early working years.)
....
....
....

(If applicable:) Are you a good manager? Give an example of a managerial accomplishment.
....
....
....

Here are a few more. Prepare answers to all of those you might be asked.
- What do you see as the most difficult task in being a manager?
- Why are you leaving your present job? (Do not lie if you've been fired, but do put the best face on it. Do not complain, accuse, or bad-mouth your previous employer. Treat your last job as a learning experience.)
- What are the five most significant accomplishments in your career so far? In your last position?
- What are your strong points?
- What are your weak points? (No one is perfect. The trick is to identify weaknesses you are aware of that you are attempting to eliminate.)
- If you could start your working career over again, what would you do differently? (Honesty is important here, as long as you still want to do the job for which you are applying.)

View the interview as a meeting between two equals—a buyer and a seller—to explore what each has to offer the other. If you convey the impression early that you have something the company wants, you will establish parity in a hurry. Listen to the questions behind the questions. For example:

"How would you evaluate your last employer?" (Any traces of vindictiveness or self pity? Any sense of not taking responsibility for your actions or decisions?)

Or

"Who was your best boss? Describe him/her." (In what kind of working environment is this person most comfortable? What tendencies might there be regarding loyalty, self-starting, working independently, or "coattailing"?)

Asking Your Own Questions

Never take the position that interviewing protocol puts all questions in the hands of the interviewer until the end of the discussion. Think of every possible aspect of the job you want to know about, every aspect of the target employer you want to know about, and every aspect of your prospective boss's background and management style you want to know about. Have your questions prepared accordingly. At appropriate times during the interview, answer the question directed at you and follow up with a question of your own on the same topic. For example:

"So the strategic plan I initiated for the trauma program effectively addressed personnel, administrative, and financial management practices. It sounds as though some of these same issues might apply to your emergency services delivery needs. Is this true?" (Such a question categorizes you immediately as a problem solver. The interviewer's response will tell you more about the situation and your potential role in it.)

Another possibility: "How would you describe the 'culture' of this organization?" (Follow-up questions to a "What do you mean?" response might be: "How do decisions get made?"; "How is excellent performance rewarded?"; "What kinds of things get people into trouble here?" and the like.)

Make the most of these serendipitous opportunities.

Interview Wrap-Up

Much can depend on how you play the interview endgame. Remember, this is your last opportunity to nail down the job offer, if you sense you are getting close. It is also a chance to resurrect your candidacy if you think an earlier blunder has damaged you.

When you feel that the interview is coming to a close ("Any further questions?" "Well, I guess that covers everything."), go out in as strong a position as you can. This is your chance to ask all of the questions you have not gotten to earlier. The response to one of them, if you have not established it previously, should include a clear awareness of the kind of person your prospective boss is looking for.

If you want the job, ask for it. Restate your understanding of the requirements and your ability to meet them. Ask a final question designed to assess or crystalize your candidacy. ("Where do you think we stand?"; "What's the next step?"; "How soon will you be making a decision?")

You have done all you can. Thank the interviewer for his or her time, and leave.

You have two final responsibilities after you leave the interview. First is to find a quiet place and record your impressions, as completely as possible. Describe any additional job requirements you discovered, as well as the extent to which you conveyed your ability to perform them. Jot down all other information that was new to you, plus any changes—for better or worse—that altered your perspective of the opportunity. Finally, write down all job-related questions yet to be answered.

Your second responsibility is to write a follow-up letter to the interviewer, as a way of (1) indicating your continued interest, (2) offering any additional reasons for you to be hired, and (3) resurrecting any "soft spots" in the interview to correct a misimpression. The sample follow-up letter on page 280 continues the job search of the cardiology nurse whose résumé and cover letter appear on pages 196 and 175, respectively. Notice that although Ms. Berrian felt that the interview went well, she takes the additional precaution of asking for any possible negative feedback. This will give her the opportunity to deal head-on with any objections Dr. Insull may have to her candidacy, and to neutralize them.

129 McLeigh Avenue
Englewood, CO 80110
February 10, 1997

Dr. Samuel Insull III
Director of Internal Medicine
Swedish Medical Center
501 E. Hampden Avenue
Englewood, CO 80110

Dear Dr. Insull:

Thanks very much for your time yesterday describing the various duties to be assumed by the cardiology/research nurse candidate you select. I particularly appreciated your thoroughness outlining the ways this position relates to the Internal Medicine Department's mission, as well as to that of the Medical Center itself.

As I mentioned, this is a job I believe I could do well, and similar to two that I *have* done well. From your description of specific duties, it would seem that the patient follow-up and research protocols I established for the VA cardiology consult and angioplasty clinics would contribute significantly to your current needs.

I view this opportunity as ideal—both for the background I am able to bring to it, and the degree to which I can help you accomplish your objectives. If you doubt my ability to perform any aspect of this job to your complete satisfaction, please let me know and I will address it specifically. I look forward to continuing our dialogue.

Sincerely,

Cassandra Berrian

Cassandra Berrian

An alternative, if you feel comfortable with it, is to follow up with a phone call. This can be more effective than a letter, but it presupposes your ability to think nimbly and to field—to the interviewer's satisfaction—any additional, off-the-wall questions he or she may ask.

THE SECOND INTERVIEW

Your invitation for a second interview confirms that you have impressed the employer with your ability to do the job. Your competition probably has been narrowed to from one to five other candidates. Presumably you have by this time a good enough reading of your prospective boss's personality and way of viewing the job to know how to elevate your candidacy and give yourself the best chance of getting the job offer.

Think of the things that got you this far in the first place and seemed to make the most favorable impact. Conversely, try to think of reasons you weren't offered the job immediately after the first interview.

Prepare for your second interview as follows: After reviewing your notes from the first interview, make two exhaustive three-column lists. For the first list, record all of your qualifications for the job in **Column A**. In **Column B**, list the degree to which you were able to articulate these qualifications to the interviewer. **Column C** will consist of the selling job that remains in the second interview, that is, A minus B.

The second list will include specific qualifications required or desired for the position that you do not have, along with any gray areas that represent conceivable negatives in your candidacy. Catalog these in **Column A**, by category. In **Column B**, record how well you handled these deficiencies and liabilities in the first interview; and in **Column C** (again, A minus B), detail the work to be done in the second interview. The lists will look like this:

ASSETS

Column A	Column B	Column C
My Qualifications	Extent Covered Previously	Points Yet to Be Made

LIABILITIES

Column A	Column B	Column C
Deficiencies/Liabilities	How Well Handled Previously	How I Will Overcome

In applying these data and conclusions to the interview itself, it is essential to strike a proper balance. Oversell—either by way of reinforcing positives or eliminating negatives—can lead to an appearance of anxiety at one extreme or defensiveness at the other. Either could be a knockout factor in receiving a job offer. It is enough to be on top of the situation, determining what issues are yet a concern, and then deal with them in a straightforward, confident manner.

Sometimes an interviewer will conclude that a candidate is unfit based on inference rather than accurate data. (This is more likely to occur in unstructured interviews.) If you feel an unease about your candidacy even though all indications point to a good fit, you have nothing to lose by forcing the issue with a question such as: "From our previous discussion, it seems to me that this is a job I could do well. Do you agree?" Anything other than emphatic agreement should be followed up aggressively. For example: "Is there anything specifically that makes you think I am not the right person for the job?" If you get an honest answer, at least you will be able to deal directly with it. If not, at least you have tried to force the issue to the best of your ability.

Finally—and be careful with this suggestion, because it does involve some risk—consider seizing the opportunity and putting some distance between you and your competitors, as follows: If you are dealing with an open, pragmatic, forceful individual, see how quickly you can get to the heart of the matter in a way that will increase the regard in which you are held.

A possible interview opener for such a person might be: "Well, what can I do to convince you that I'm the best person for this job?" or (perhaps with a slight smile), "What is preventing you from offering me the job right now?" This forcing style, consistent with the personality of the interviewer, may help you be seen as an assertive, contributing department member. (Surgeons, pathologists, physician's assistants, and others who find a decisive personality an asset, may consider this an ideal way to project a persona the interviewer was about to probe for anyway.)

Be sure you have gauged your interviewer carefully, though. A more reflective, controlled interviewer will surely judge such a question to be boorish or otherwise inappropriate, enough to knock you out of the running.

NEGOTIATING COMPENSATION

Those of you changing careers or entering the job market straight from school probably will not have much negotiating leeway. Without previous experience or a list of accomplishments as leverage, your power to influence the salary and benefits package offered you is virtually nil. What you can do—in fact, should do—is find out how the employer rewards good performance. You must be comfortable with the way you will be treated six months or a year from now if you do everything expected of you, and do it in exemplary fashion. Ask for chapter and verse on the institution's raise and promotion policy.

Those of you with a good track record should exploit previous accomplishments as much as possible, and determine if the employer wants you badly enough to modify its opening offer. You won't be criticized for trying to improve your position if your request is made in a relatively low-key manner. And even if this does not work, at least you won't be bitter about not having tried at all. If you feel uneasy about negotiating the terms of your employment, read John Tarrant's *Perks and Parachutes* (Simon & Schuster, 1985) to get some sound bargaining-table psychology and strategy, including copies of actual employment contracts, with terms.

TAKING YOUR NEW-JOB PULSE

Get in the habit of monitoring your performance, beginning your first day on the new job. Don't just keep track of successful assignments; evaluate your relationships with the people around you: subordinates, peers, and supervisors. Learn to assess your ability and willingness to anticipate and solve those problems within your sphere of influence. Also:

- Ask for feedback. Colleagues you trust see things you do not. Find a time to ask your boss "How'm I doing?" occasionally—meaning well before your review date, so if corrective action is indicated, you can do what you have to do.
- Record your accomplishments. Make a copy of every good report, proposal, or completed project that led to a solved problem, departmental or institutional growth, or reduced expenses.
- Spread your wings. Broaden and enrich your professional reputation by getting involved in your specialty's state, regional, and national organizations. Become active; volunteer for assignments at workshops, seminars, and meetings.
- Look for opportunities. After a year or two on your new job, an opening may occur elsewhere in the organization more consistent with your talents and long-term career goals. *Follow organizational procedure to the letter* (to be sure your ambition is not interpreted, to your peril, as dissatisfaction with your current assignment—or boss!). Then use the interviewing skills learned in this book to improve your chances.

  Treat the new opportunity as you would an opening elsewhere. Many fail to realize they may be competing with excellent candidates outside the company, and proceed as though their performance record and inside status automatically gives them a decisive edge. It does not. Those who realize this have the best chance for success.

Good luck with your job search, and with the new job you find as a result.

Bibliography

The following books and directories are intended to provide job-search or career-change assistance of three different kinds:
1) Information or source material for individual healthcare occupations, or clusters of occupations
2) Generic job-search strategy or advice transcending specific occupations or specialties
3) Scholarship, grant, and low-cost loan sources

Suggestion: Skim entries one perspective at a time, starting with your highest priority, to target possible useful source material. When one area of research is complete, run through the next list to illuminate your second focus of interest; then the third.

HEALTHCARE INDUSTRY INFORMATION SOURCES

Allied Health and Rehabilitation Professions Education Directory (1996–1997 Edition). Chicago: American Medical Association, 1996. Listings of accredited educational programs for 36 allied health occupations. Divided into four sections: (1) information on eight accrediting agencies; (2) occupational descriptions and complete list of educational programs by state, including certification, licensure, and registration; (3) names and addresses of 2,000 institutions (schools, hospitals, and medical centers) sponsoring more than 3,000 accredited professional health education programs; (4) tables and charts of graduation, enrollment, and attrition data by state and specialty.

Cambridge Educational Catalog, multiple series of healthcare career videos: "School to Work," "Day in a Career," "Enter Here," "Career Encounters," "Vocational Visions." Write Cambridge Educational for a catalog at P.O. Box 2153, Charleston, WV 25328; or call (800) 468-4227. (Some titles may be available for loan or rental at your local library.)

The Career Guide, Dun's Employment Opportunities Directory, 1996. Bethlehem, PA: Dun & Bradstreet Information Services, 1995. A professional employment guide providing comprehensive coverage on employers. Includes allied health, nursing, pharmacy, and hospitals. Describes disciplines hired, career opportunities, training and development, benefits, etc.

Damp, Dennis, *The Book of U.S. Government Jobs: Where They Are, What's Available, and How to Get One.* Moon Township, PA: Bookhaven Press, 1996. Practical advice on gaining access to the thousands of new jobs available annually in VA hospitals, outpatient clinics, and government-run nursing homes from entry level to professional occupations throughout the United States.

Damp, Dennis, *The Health Care Job Explosion! Careers in the 90's.* Moon Township, PA: Bookhaven Press, 1993. Includes projections and statistics in allied health occupations across the board.

Dun's Healthcare Reference Book. Bethlehem, PA: Dun & Bradstreet, 1995. More than 30,000 healthcare businesses and institutions, listed alphabetically, geographically, and by industry. For suppliers: names, addresses, phone numbers, and products and services specialized. For providers (e.g., hospitals): number of beds, number of physicians, number and kinds of nurses, population served. Similar information for labs, home health agencies, hospices, long-term care facilities, and occupational and physical therapy facilities.

Guide to Nursing Programs. Princeton, NJ: Peterson's Guides, 1994. Provides information on more than 1,500 baccalaurate and graduate nursing programs at over 600 schools. Gives sources for financial aid and top job locations. Published in cooperation with the American Association of Colleges for Nursing.

Graduate Medical Education Directory (1995–1996). Chicago: American Medical Association, 1995. Official list of programs accredited by the Accreditation Council for Graduate Medical Education. Provides medical students with residency information regarding requirements for licensure, certification, and the Match; features program listings for more than 7,600 residency and fellowship programs by specialty and subspecialty, city and state.

Graduate Programs in Business, Education, Health and Law. Princeton, NJ: Peterson's Guides, 1996. Volume 6 provides wide-ranging information on graduate and professional healthcare programs in the United States, Canada, Mexico, Europe, and Africa. Capsule summaries of programs, in addition to one- or two-page descriptions of the institutions. Includes programs of study, research facilities, financial aid, costs, and application procedures. (Visit Peterson's Education Center on the Internet: http://www.petersons.com)

Harkavy, Michael, *101 Careers: A Guide to the Fastest-Growing Opportunities.* New York: John Wiley & Sons, Inc., 1990. Twenty-eight of them are in the healthcare field, all categorized by job description, prospects, qualifications, personal skills, and earnings. Double check with a more recent source (such as *Your Career in Healthcare*) to incorporate the most up-to-date research.

The Health Care Almanac. Chicago: American Medical Association, 1995. Comprehensive, instructive, and entertaining. Defines and analyzes medical issues and terms from acupuncture to managed care. Effectively combines quoted reference material, cogent definitions, and provocative points of view with whimsy, poetry, and unconventional observations.

Healthcare Reference Book, 1995/96. Bethlehem, PA: Dun & Bradstreet. Provides information on the more than 30,000 businesses and institutions that make up America's healthcare industry. Includes S.I.C. Codes. Covers hospitals, pharmaceutical companies, laboratories, medical device manufacturers, etc.

Job Opportunities in Health Care. Princeton, NJ: Peterson's Guides, 1994. Listings for more than 1,500 healthcare companies, including product or service specialization, addresses and phone numbers, and "expertise needed" entry. (Take the latter with a grain of salt until you investigate on your own. Also, research and write your "prospective boss"; not the human resource contact listed.)

McPhee, John, *Heirs of General Practice.* New York: Farrar, Straus, Giroux, 1984. For those of you considering medical school but who are ambivalent about specializing or pursuing general practice, McPhee puts the case in his customary thorough, sensitive fashion.

A Medical Student's Guide to Strolling Through the Match. Kansas City, MO, American Academy of Family Physicians (undated). The subtitle tells it all: "The What, Where, When, Why, & How of Residency Selection." Assists medical students in the decision-making process at various stages—choosing a specialty, preparing a C.V., selecting residency programs, interviewing tips, and bibliography.

Swanson, Barbara, *Careers in Health Care.* Lincolnwood, IL: NTC Publishing Group, 1994. Descriptions of 58 allied health and related healthcare service occupations, consisting of educational requirements, job descriptions, expected remuneration and career paths.

GENERIC JOB-SEARCH STRATEGY AND ADVICE

Criscito, Pat, *Designing the Perfect Résumé.* Hauppauge, NY: Barron's Educational Series, 1995. How to use a home computer to design a professional-looking résumé. Hundreds of sample résumés created with WordPerfect software. Includes practical details such as effective use of layout, section heads, type fonts, bullets, and graphic devices. Tips on designing effective letterheads and cover letters, as well.

Crowther, Karmen, *Researching Your Way to a Good Job.* New York: John Wiley & Sons, 1993. Provides tools and techniques to examine potential employers and jobs, and job-related information on other communities, if you intend to relocate.

Encyclopedia of Associations, 1995 Edition. Detroit: Gale Research, Inc., 1994. More than 22,000 national and international organizations, listed alphabetically, many of them in the healthcare industry. Provides such information as number of members, budget, publications, purpose, and mission. To indicate the level of specialty represented, you will find everything from the Association of Nurses in AIDS Care to the International Society of the Knee.

Internet Yellow Pages, 1996 Edition. Berkeley, CA: Osborne/McGraw-Hill. A user-friendly guide to the Internet. Several pages related to healthcare, including newsgroups, information, discussion clubs, research, etc. Good networking source.

Levine, John R., Carol Baroudi, Margaret Levine Young, *The Internet for Dummies, 3rd Edition.* Foster City, CA: IDG Books Worldwide, Inc., 1995. An articulate guide for getting on the net, getting to where you want to go, and for using e-mail, software, newsgroups, and so on.

Occupational Outlook Handbook. Washington, D.C.: U.S. Department of Labor, Bureau of Labor Statistics (1996–1997 Edition). A nationally recognized source of career information for nearly 50 years. Describes what workers do on the job, the training and education needed, earnings, working conditions, and job prospects covering hundreds of healthcare jobs in most diagnostic, assessment, treatment, technical, and service occupations.

Professional and Occupational Licensing Directory. Detroit: Gale Research, Inc., 1993. Provides detailed information on all licenses required for a specific occupation, including more than 1,000 state and federal agencies and boards.

Strunk, William, Jr., and E.B. White, *Elements of Style.* 3rd ed. New York: Macmillan Publishing Co., Inc., 1979. The best book in print on making words count.

Vincent, Patrick, *Free Stuff on the Internet.* Scottsdale, AZ: Coriolis Group, 1995. In addition to the downloadable goodies, dozens of job-search sources—among them Overseas Jobs, Internetworking, Career Connection's Online Information, and Online Career Center.

Vocational Careers Sourcebook. Detroit: Gale Research, Inc., 1992. Provides a broad spectrum of available information on vocational career opportunities, including guides to send for, associations, certification, periodicals, and other source information.

Wilson, Robert F. *Conducting Better Job Interviews.* Hauppauge, NY: Barron's Educational Series, 1991. Secrets from the other side of the desk. What new managers are taught about how to choose the best person for the job.

Wilson, Robert F. and Erik Rambusch, *Conquering Résumé Objections* and *Conquering Interview Objections.* New York: John Wiley & Sons, 1994. "The résumé book includes a gem of a chapter on before-and-after resumé samples," writes James Gallagher in the International Association of Career Management Professionals newsletter. "The second volume on interviewing fills the missing link with everything you need to know about strategy, preparation, presentation, and follow-up for your job-campaign interviews."

Wilson, Robert F., *Interview to Win Your First Job.* New Haven: Wilson McLeran, Inc., 1996 (Second Edition). Video and workbook program for high school and college students preparing for their first full-time, permanent job search. (". . . probably the best tape on the subject this reviewer has seen." —*The Library Journal.*)

Zinsser, William, *On Writing Well.* New York: HarperCollins Publishers, 1990. Sound advice for anyone utilizing the written word. Dozens of examples of good writing, buttressed by sound analysis.

SCHOLARSHIP, GRANT, AND LOW-COST LOAN SOURCES

Health Education Assistance Loan (HEAL) Program. A federally insured loan program for eligible graduate students in schools of medicine, osteopathy, dentistry, veterinary medicine, optometry, podiatry, public health, pharmacy, chiropractic, or in programs in health administration and clinical psychology. Under the terms of this program, students may borrow up to $20,000 per year (some specialties award $12,500 per year) for tuition, fees, books, supplies and equipment, lab expenses, and living expenses. Details available at the financial aid office of all participating schools.

Scholarships & Loans for Nursing Education, 1995–1996. New York: National League for Nursing, 1995. Includes everything from choosing a school to the range of federal, state, and "other" sources for scholarships, grants, and loans. Special sections on aid for minority students, post-doctoral study, and research grants.

Paying Less for College, 1996. Princeton, NJ: Peterson's Guides, Princeton, New Jersey, 1995. Comprehensive guide to the more than $36 billion awarded annually in institutional, private, state, and federal aid; 1,600+ college financial aid profiles and cost comparisons "not found elsewhere," reads the back-cover blurb. Explains the new-for-1997 financial aid application process. Indexes of colleges offering scholarships for athletics, academics, civic or religious service, and ethnic and religious background.

Schlachter, Gail Ann and R. David Weber, *Directory of Financial Aids for Minorities, 1995–97.* San Carlos, CA: Reference Services Press. Contains 2,014 references, 550 sources: government agencies, private organizations, corporations, sororities and fraternities, foundations, religious groups, and military and veterans' associations providing assistance, either exclusively or primarily for minorities. The inside story on eligibility; number, amount, and kind of assistance awarded (and for how long); how, where, and when to apply; what limitations might be applicable.

Need a Lift. The American Legion. Details on the various programs this veterans' organization sponsors on behalf of needy students. (Similar programs available from such civic groups as the YMCA, 4-H Club, Elks, Kiwanis, Jaycees, Chamber of Commerce, the Girl Scouts, and the Boy Scouts.)

Student Guide to Federal Financial Aid Programs, 1996–97. User-friendly handbook through the maze of government assistance to higher education. Begins by mentioning complementary and supplementary sources at state level, in addition to other public and private sources. Explanations of every available grant and loan (including loans to parents)—contingencies, qualifications, deadlines, special circumstances that may affect eligibility, payback schedules, and list of important terms and concepts to understand. For a free copy, write Federal Aid Information Center, P.O. Box 84, Washington, D.C. 20044–0084; or call (800) 433-3243. (The student guide is also available online, on the Department of Education's World Wide Web site, through the Internet. The site address is: http://www.ed.gov)

APPENDIX A

Glossary of Basic Healthcare Terms and Abbreviations

A.A.F.P.   American Academy of Family Physicians

A.A.M.A.   American Association of Medical Assistants

A.A.P.   American Academy of Pediatrics; American Association of Pathologists

A.A.P.S.   American Academy of Plastic Surgeons

A.C.C.   American College of Cardiology

A.C.E.P.   American College of Emergency Physicians

A.C.N.M.   American College of Nurse-Midwives

A.C.O.G.   American College of Obstetricians and Gynecologists

A.C.P.   American College of Pathologists

Acquired Immunodeficiency Syndrome (AIDS)   end-stage manifestation of a prolonged, chronic erosion of the immune system caused by the human immunodeficiency virus (HIV)

acupuncture   insertion of stainless steel needles into various body locations, used in treating certain disorders

allied health   health-related personnel who fulfill necessary roles in the healthcare system, complementing the work of physicians and other healthcare specialists

A.M.A.   American Medical Association

anesthesiologist   a physician specializing in anesthesiology

anesthetic   a drug or agent used to eliminate the sensation of pain

anesthetist   a person, such as a nurse or technician, trained to administer anesthetics

A.O.A.   American Optometric Association; American Osteopathic Association

A.O.R.N.   American Organization of Registered Nurses

A.P.H.A.   American Public Health Association

A.S.C.L.T.   American Society of Clinical Laboratory Technicians

A.S.C.P.   American Society of Clinical Pathologists

audiologist   a person skilled in audiology, including the rehabilitation of those whose impaired hearing cannot be improved by medical or surgical means

audiology the science of hearing, particularly the study of impaired hearing that cannot be improved by medication or surgical therapy

audiometry measurement of hearing, as by means of an audiometer

biomedical biological and medical; pertaining to the application of natural sciences (e.g., biology, biochemistry, biophysics) to the study of medicine

biomedicine clinical medicine based on the principles of the natural sciences (e.g., biology, biochemistry, biophysics)

biopsy the removal and examination, usually microscopic, of living body tissue, performed to establish precise diagnosis

C.A.D.A.C Certified Alcohol and Drug Abuse Counselor

cadaver a dead body; generally applied to a human body preserved for anatomical study

C.A.H.E.A. Committee on Allied Health Education and Accreditation

C.A.P. College of American Pathologists

cardiac pertaining to the heart

cardiologist a physician skilled in the diagnosis and treatment of heart disease

cardiology the study of the heart and its functions

C.A.T. computerized axial tomography

C.D.C. Centers for Disease Control

clinical medicine the study of disease by direct examination of the living patient

clinical nurse specialist a registered nurse with a high degree of knowledge, skill, and competence in a specialized area of nursing

C.M.A. Certified Medical Assistant

C.P.H. certificate in public health

C.R.N.A. Certified Registered Nurse Anesthetist

C.T. computerized tomography (also C.A.T.: computerized axial tomography)

culture cultivation of living organisms in special material to encourage their growth

cytology study of the structure and function of cells

cytotechnologist technologist trained to work with pathologists to detect changes in body cells that may be important in the early diagnosis of cancer and other diseases

D.D.S. Doctor of Dental Surgery

dental hygienist auxiliary member of the dental profession trained in the art of removing calcareous deposits and stains from the surfaces of the teeth, and in providing information on the prevention of oral disease and other services

dentistry 1. department of the healing arts concerned with the teeth, oral cavity, and associated structures, including the diagnosis and treatment of their diseases and the restoration of defective and missing tissue; 2. the work done by dentists, such as the creation of restorations, crowns, and bridges, as well as surgical procedures performed in and about the oral cavity

dermatologist a physician whose practice is limited to the diagnosis and treatment of skin disorders

dermatology medical specialty concerned with the diagnosis and treatment of skin disorders

D.M.D. Doctor of Dental Medicine

D.V.M. Doctor of Veterinary Medicine (also V.M.D.)

echocardiography ultrasound procedure to monitor heart rhythm, used by physicians in the diagnosis of heart disease and the study of the heart

E.E.G. electroencephalogram: a recording of electrical energy on the skull generated by currents emanating spontaneously from nerve cells in the brain

E.K.G. (also E.C.G.) electrocardiogram: a recording of the changes of electrical energy occurring during the heartbeat (used especially in diagnosing abnormalities of heart action)

electroneurodiagnostic technology scientific field devoted to recording and studying the electrical activity of the brain and nervous system

E.N.T. Ear, Nose, and Throat

family physician a medical specialist who plans and provides the comprehensive primary healthcare of all members of a family, regardless of age or sex, on a continuing basis

gastroenterologist a physician who specializes in diseases of the digestive tract

gastroenterology the study of the stomach and intestines and their diseases

geriatrics branch of medicine dealing with problems of old age and aged people

gerontology branch of knowledge dealing with aging and the problems of the aged

health maintenance organization (HMO) organization responsible for both financing and providing an agreed-upon set of health maintenance and treatment services to a specifically defined population for a prepaid, fixed sum

hematologist a specialist in the study of the blood

hematology branch of medical science that treats the form and structure of blood and blood-forming tissues

histology department of anatomy that deals with the minute structure, composition, and function of tissues; also called microscopical anatomy

histopathology the histology of diseased tissues

HIV human immunodeficiency virus

holistic medicine form of therapy treating the whole person, not just the part or parts in which symptoms occur

homeopathic medicine a system of alternative medicine that seeks to treat patients by administering small doses of substances that would bring on symptoms similar to those of the patient in a healthy person

I.C.S. International College of Surgeons

immunology branch of biomedical science concerned with the phenomena and causes of immunity

internal medicine branch of medicine that deals with the diagnosis and treatment of diseases and injuries of human internal organ systems

locum tenens physicians who hold positions for other physicians when they must be absent from their practices

L.P.N. licensed practical nurse

managed care systems used to affect access to and control payment for healthcare services

Medicaid a medical assistance program jointly financed by state and federal governments for eligible low-income individuals

Medicare a federally-funded health insurance program providing coverage for people aged 65 or older, younger people receiving social security disability benefits, and people who need dialysis or kidney transplants

M.P.H.   Master of Public Health

M.R.A.   medical record administrator

M.R.I.   magnetic resonance imaging

M.S.W.   Master of Social Work

myopathy   any disease of a muscle

N.A.E.M.T.   National Association of Emergency Medical Technicians

N.B.M.E.   National Board of Medical Examiners

N.C.I.   National Cancer Institute

neuralgia   paroxysmal pain that extends along the course of one or more nerves

neurologist   an expert in neurology or in the treatment of disorders of the nervous system

neurology   branch of medical science that deals with the nervous system, both normal and in disease; clinical neurology is that specialty concerned with the diagnosis and treatment of disorders of the nervous system

neurosurgeon   a physician who specializes in neurosurgery

neurosurgery   surgery of the nervous system designed to restore normal conductivity in malfunctional nerve fibers or to improve blood flow in nerve tissue

N.I.H.   National Institutes of Health, the principal biomedical research agency of the federal government

N.I.M.H.   National Institute of Mental Health

nuclear medicine   medical specialty that uses the nuclear properties of radioactive and stable nuclides to make diagnostic evaluations of the body and provide therapy with radioactive sources

obstetrician   a physician who specializes in the treatment of women before, during, and after childbirth

oncology   the body of knowledge concerning tumors; the study of tumors

O.S.H.A.   Occupational Safety and Health Administration

ophthalmologist   a physician who specializes in the diagnosis and medical and surgical treatment of diseases and defects of the eye and related structures

ophthalmology   branch of medicine dealing with the eye, its anatomy, physiology, and pathology

orthodontics   branch of dentistry that deals with the development, prevention, and correction of irregularities of the teeth and malocclusion and with associated facial abnormalities

orthopedics   branch of surgery specially concerned with the preservation and restoration of the function of the skeletal system, its articulations and associated structures

orthopedist   a physician who specializes in orthopedics

osteopathic medicine   a system of therapy based on the theory that the body is capable of making its own remedies against disease and other toxic conditions when it is in normal structural relationship and has favorable environmental conditions and adequate nutrition

otolaryngology   branch of medicine diagnosing and treating diseases of the ear, nose, and throat

pathology   1. branch of medicine that studies the essential nature of disease, especially the structural and functional changes in tissues and organs of the body that cause or are caused by disease; 2. the structural and functional manifestations of disease

pediatrics   branch of medicine diagnosing and treating diseases and injuries to children from birth through adolescence

perfusionist technologist skilled in operating equipment to temporarily replace a patient's circulatory or respiratory function

periodontal situated or occurring around a tooth; pertaining to the periodontium

periodontics branch of dentistry dealing with the study and treatment of diseases of the periodontium

pharmacist one licensed to prepare and sell or dispense drugs and compounds and to make up prescriptions; an apothecary or druggist

pharmacology science that deals with the origin, nature, chemistry, effects, and uses of drugs

Pharm.D Doctor of Pharmacy

phlebotomy incision of a vein for purposes of collecting and analyzing blood

physiatrist a physician who specializes in the use of physical devices and exercise to rehabilitate patients

physician authorized practitioner of medicine, graduated from a college of medicine or osteopathy and licensed by the appropriate governing board

physician assistant one trained in an accredited program and certified by a board to perform certain of a physician's duties under the supervision of a licensed physician

podiatry the specialized field that deals with the study and care of the foot, including its anatomy, pathology, and medical and surgical treatment

primary care area of medical practice combining branches of family practice, internal medicine, pediatrics, and obstetrics/gynecology

proctologist a physician who specializes in the treatment of diseases and disorders of the anus, rectum, and colon

psychiatry branch of medicine that deals with the study, treatment, and prevention of mental illness

psychotherapy treatment designed to produce a response by mental rather than by physical effects, including the use of suggestion, reeducation, reassurance, and support, as well as the techniques of hypnosis and psychoanalysis

psychotropic exerting an effect upon the mind; capable of modifying mental activity, usually applied to drugs that affect the mental state

radiologist a physician who specializes in the use of radiant energy (e.g., x-rays) in the diagnosis and treatment of disease

radiology the science of radiant energy and radiant substances, especially that branch of the health sciences that deals with the use of radiant energy in the diagnosis and treatment of disease

relapse the return of a disease after its apparent cessation

renal pertaining to the kidney

retinopathy any noninflammatory disease of the retina

R.N. registered nurse

Roentgen, Wilhelm Conrad German physicist, 1845–1923, who discovered roentgen rays (the international unit of x or y radiation) in 1895; winner of 1901 Nobel prize in physics

roentgenogram a film produced by roentgenography

seroconversion the development of antibodies in response to infection or administration of a vaccine

seroculture   a bacterial culture or blood serum

serology   the study of antigen-antibody reactions in an artificial environment

serotype   the type of microorganism as determined by the kinds and combinations of antigens present in the cell

side effect   a consequence other than the one(s) for which an agent or measure is used, as the adverse effects produced by a drug, especially on a tissue or organ system other than the one sought to be benefited by its administration

sonogram   a record or display obtained by ultrasonic scanning

sonographer   diagnostician who uses medical ultrasound under the supervision of a physician for the use and interpretation of ultrasound procedures

synergist   a medicine that aids or cooperates with another

synergy   correlated action or cooperation on the part of two or more structures or drugs; in neurology, the faculty by which movements are properly grouped for the peformance of acts requiring special adjustments

T.B.   tuberculosis

therapist   a person skilled in the treatment of disease; often combined with a term indicating the specific type of disorder treated (as speech therapist) or a particular type of treatment rendered (as physical therapist)

tomograph   an apparatus for moving an x-ray source in one direction as the film is moved in the opposite direction

tomography   the recording of internal body images at a predetermined plane by means of a tomograph

ultrasonography   the visualization of deep structures of the body by recording the reflections (echoes) of pulses of ultrasonic waves directed into the tissues; also called echography and sonography

urology   branch of medicine concerned with male and female urinary tracts, and with male genital organs

venipuncture   puncture of a vein

vessel   any channel for carrying a fluid, such as the blood or lymph

water-borne   propagated by contaminated drinking water; said of diseases

W.H.O.   World Health Organization, an international agency associated with the United Nations

zoology   the biology of animals

APPENDIX B

Healthcare Positions by SOC Numbers

In the following list of occupations covered in *Your Career in Healthcare,* the column headed "SOC" indicates specific Standard Occupational Classification code numbers designated by the U.S. Department of Labor Bureau of Labor Statistics, and correlated accordingly in the Bureau's *Occupational Outlook Handbook.* The column headed "D.O.T. Title" lists Dictionary of Occupational Titles allocated to respective SOC numbers, for ready reference when using the *Handbook.*

SOC	D.O.T. Title	SOC	D.O.T. Title
1310	Emergency medical services coordinator	2610	Dermatologist
		2610	Family practitioner
1310	Medical record administrator	2610	General practitioner
1854	Cytologist	2610	Gynecologist
1854	Geneticist	2610	Internist
1854	Physiologist	2610	Public health physician
1855	Public-health microbiologist	2610	Neurologist
1915	Psychologist, clinical	2610	Obstetrician
1915	Psychologist, counseling	2610	Ophthalmologist
1915	Psychologist, educational	2610	Otolaryngologist
1915	Psychologist, social	2610	Pediatrician
2032	Social worker, medical	2610	Physiatrist
2032	Social worker, psychiatric	2610	Proctologist
2032	Substance abuse counselor	2610	Radiologist
2400	Counselor, nurses association	2610	Surgeon
2610	Pathologist	2610	Urologist
2610	Anesthesiologist	2610	Psychiatrist
2610	Cardiologist	2610	Osteopathic physician

SOC	D.O.T. Title	SOC	D.O.T. Title
2620	Dentist	3620	Cytogenic technologist
2620	Endodontist	3620	Cytotechnologist
2620	Oral and maxillofacial surgeon	3620	Medical technologist
2620	Orthodontist	3630	Dental technician
2620	Pediatric dentist	3640	Medical record technician
2620	Periodontist	3650	Nuclear medicine technologist
2620	Prosthodontist	3650	Radiation-therapy technologist
2620	Public-health dentist	3650	Radiologic technologist
2700	Veterinarian	3650	Special procedures technologist, cardiac catheterization
2810	Optometrist		
2830	Podiatrist	3650	Special procedures technologist, CAT scan
2890	Chiropractor		
2900	Nurse anesthetist	3650	Special procedures technologist, magnetic resonance imaging (MRI)
2900	Nurse executive		
2900	Nurse, general duty	3660	Nurse, licensed practical
2900	Nurse, head	3690	Holter scanning technician
2900	Nurse-midwife	3690	Ophthalmic technician
2900	Nurse practitioner	3690	Optometric assistant
2900	Nurse, staff	3690	Electrocardiograph technician
2900	Nurse, supervisor	3690	Electroencephalographic technologist
3010	Pharmacist	3690	Cardiopulmonary technologist
3020	Dietitian, research	3690	Paramedic
3020	Dietitian, chief	3690	Emergency medical technician
3020	Dietitian, clinical	3690	Stress test technician
3020	Dietitian, community	3690	Ultrasound technologist
3020	Dietitian, consultant	3690	Echocardiograph technician
3020	Dietitian, teaching	3690	Surgical technician
3031	Respiratory therapist	4490	Optician, dispensing
3032	Occupational therapist	4490	Optician apprentice, dispensing
3032	Physical therapist	5232	Dental assistant
3034	Audiologist	5233	Medical assistant
3034	Speech pathologist	5236	Nursing aide
3039	Dance therapist	5236	Psychiatric aide
3040	Physician assistant	5624	Animal attendant
3620	Biochemistry technologist	6865	Dental laboratory technician
3620	Microbiology technologist		

APPENDIX C

Healthcare-Related Associations

Accreditation Review Committee for the
   Anesthesiologist's Assistant
515 N. State Street, Suite 7530
Chicago, IL 60610
(accreditation information)

American Academy of Anesthesiologists'
   Assistants
P.O. Box 33876
Decatur, GA 30033
(curriculum and career information)

American Academy of Family Physicians
8880 Ward Parkway
Kansas City, MO 64114
(general information)

American Academy of Ophthalmology
655 Beach Street
San Francisco, CA 94120
(general information)

American Academy of Physician Assistants
950 N. Washington Street
Alexandria, VA 22314
(career information)

American Art Therapy Association, Inc.
1202 Allanson Road
Mundelein, IL 60060

American Association of Blood Banks
8101 Glenbrook Road
Bethesda, MD 20814
(accreditation, career and curriculum
   information)

American Association of Colleges of Nursing
1 DuPont Circle, Suite 530
Washington, DC 20036
(list of B.S. nursing and graduate programs)

American Association of Colleges of
   Osteopathic Medicine
6110 Executive Boulevard, Suite 405
Rockville, MD 20852
(general career information)

American Association of Colleges of
   Pharmacy
1426 Prince Street
Alexandria, VA 22314
(career information, professional
   requirements, financial aid)

American Association of Colleges of Podiatric
   Medicine
1350 Piccard Drive, Suite 322
Rockville, MD 20850-4307
(information on colleges, requirements,
   financial aid)

American Association of Medical Assistants
20 N. Wacker Drive
Chicago, IL 60606
(general career information)

American Chiropractic Association
1701 Clarendon Boulevard
Arlington, VA 22209
(information on careers)

American Association of Dental Schools
1625 Massachusetts Avenue NW
Washington, DC 20036
(career information, list of accredited schools)

American Association for Counseling and Development
5999 Stevenson Avenue
Alexandria, VA 22304
(information on career opportunities and education)

American College of Nurse-Midwives
818 Connecticut Avenue NW, Suite 900
Washington, DC 20006
(list of accredited nurse-midwife programs)

American Dance Therapy Association, Inc.
2000 Century Plaza, Suite 108
Columbia, MD 21044
(general career information)

American Dental Assistants Association
203 LaSalle Street, Suite 1320
Chicago, IL 60601
(career information)

American Dental Hygienists' Association
Professional Development Division
444 N. Michigan Avenue, Suite 3400
(general career information)

American Dietetic Association
216 W. Jackson Boulevard, Suite 800
Chicago, IL 60606-6995
(list of academic programs, scholarships, other information)

American Health Care Association
1201 L Street NW
Washington, DC 20005-4014
(information on nursing careers in long-term care)

American Health Information Management Association
919 N. Michigan Avenue, Suite 1400
Chicago, IL 60611
(accredited medical record administrators programs information)

American Medical Association
515 N. State Street
Chicago, IL 60610
(general information)

American Nurses' Association
600 Maryland Avenue SW
Washington, DC 20024-2571
(information on career opportunities as a registered nurse)

American Occupational Therapy Association
4270 Montgomery Lane
Bethesda, MD 20824
(career information, list of educational programs)

American Optometric Association
Educational Services
243 N. Lindbergh Boulevard
St. Louis, MO 63141-7881
(career information, list of accredited schools)

American Osteopathic Association
Department of Public Relations
142 E. Ontario Street
Chicago, IL 60611
(general career information)

American Pharmaceutical Association
2215 Constitution Avenue, NW
Washington, DC 20037
(educational and financial aid information)

American Physical Therapy Association
1111 N. Fairfax Street
Alexandria, VA 22314
(career information, list of accredited educational programs)

American Podiatric Medical Association
9312 Old Georgetown Road
Bethesda, MD 20814-1621
(career information)

American Psychological Association
750 First Street, NE
Washington, DC 20005
(information on career opportunities and education)

American Registry of Diagnostic Medical Sonographers
600 Jefferson Plaza, Suite 360
Rockville, MD 20852
(certification/registration information)

American Society for Clinical Laboratory
  Sciences
7910 Woodmont Avenue, Suite 1301
Bethesda, MD 20814
(career and curriculum information)

American Society of Cardiovascular
  Professionals
120 Falcon Drive, Unit 3
Fredericksburg, VA 22408
(career and curriculum information)

American Society of Clinical Pathology
Board of Registry
P.O. Box 12277
Chicago, IL 60612-0277
(certification information)

American Society of Cytology
1015 Chestnut Street, Suite 1518
Philadelphia, PA 19107
(career information)

American Society of Echocardiography
4101 Lake Boone Trail, Suite 201
Raleigh, NC 27607
(career and curriculum information)

American Speech-Language-Hearing
  Association
10801 Rockville Pike
Rockville, MD 20852
(general information)

American Veterinary Medical Association
1931 N. Meacham Road, Suite 100
Schaumburg, IL 60173-4360
(career information for vets and vet
  technology)

Anesthesiologists' Assistant Program
Case Western University
2074 Abbington Road
Cleveland, OH 44106
(general information)

Association of American Medical Colleges
Section for Student Services
2450 N Street NW
Washington, DC 20337-1131
(list of schools, information on premed
  education, financial aid)

Association of American Veterinary Medical
  Colleges
1101 Vermont Avenue NW, Suite 710
Washington, DC 20005
(educational information)

Association of Physician Assistant Programs
950 N. Washington Street
Alexandria, VA 22314
(list of accredited programs, catalog of
  training programs)

Association of Surgical Technologists
7108-C South Alton Way
Englewood, CO 80112
(information about certification and
  accredited programs)

Cardiovascular Credentialing International
4456 Corporation Lane, Suite 120
Virginia Beach, VA 23462
(certification and registration information)

Center for Mental Health Services
Human Resource Planning and Development
  Branch
Room 15C 18
Rockville, MD 20857
(mental health workers career information)

Commission on Accreditation of Allied
  Health Education Programs
515 N. State Street, Suite 7530
Chicago, IL 60610
(accreditation information for all allied health
  programs)

Department of Veterans Affairs
Title 38 Employment Division (054D)
810 Vermont Avenue NW
Washington, DC 20420
(information about employment in VA
  medical centers)

Institute of Food Technologists
221 N. LaSalle Street
Chicago, IL 60601
(food technology and food science
  information)

Joint Review Committee for Respiratory
  Therapy Education
1701 Euless Boulevard, Suite 300
Euless, TX 76040
(list of accredited programs)

Joint Review Committee on Education in Cardiovascular Technology
911 Old Georgetown Road
Bethesda, MD 20814
(program accreditation information and arrangements for site visits)

Joint Review Committee on Education in Diagnostic Medical Sonography
20 N. Wacker Drive, Suite 900
Chicago, IL 60606
(list of accredited programs)

Joint Review Committee on Education in Radiologic Technology
20 N. Wacker Drive, Suite 900
Chicago, IL 60606
(education and credentials information)

Joint Review Committee on Educational Programs in Nuclear Medicine Technology
1144 W. 3300 South
Salt Lake City, UT 84119
(information on educational requirements)

National Accreditation Agency for Clinical Laboratory Sciences
8410 W. Bryn Mawr, Suite 670
Chicago, IL 60631
(educational and accreditation information)

National Association of Boards of Pharmacy
700 Busse Highway
Park Ridge, IL 60068
(information on licensure requirements)

National Association of Dental Laboratories
National Board for Certification in Dental Lab Technology
555 E. Braddock Road
Alexandria, VA 23314
(information about accredited training programs and certification)

National Association of Emergency Medical Technicians
102 W. Leake Street
Clinton, MS 39056
(general career information)

National Association of Social Workers, Inc.
Education Office
750 First Street NE, Suite 700
Washington, DC 20002
(medical and psychiatric social worker career information)

National Association of State Mental Health Program Directors
66 Canal Center Plaza, Suite 302
Alexandria, VA 22314
(information on respective state departments of mental health)

National Association for Music Therapy
8455 Colesville Road, Suite 930
Silver Spring, MD 20910
(career and curriculum information)

National Commission on Certification of Physician Assistants
2845 Henderson Mill Road NE
Atlanta, GA 30341
(eligibility requirements, description of certifying exam)

National Health Careers Information Hotline
Thomas Jefferson University College of Allied Sciences
Philadelphia, PA 19107
(health and mental health educational program information)

National League for Nursing
Communications Department
350 Hudson Street
New York, NY 10014
(complete list of NLS publications)

National Society for Histotechnology
4201 Northview Drive, Suite 502
Bowie, MD 20716
(career and curriculum information)

Society of Vascular Technology
4601 Presidents Drive, Suite 260
Lanham, MD 20706
(career and curriculum information)

APPENDIX D

Career Investigation

CAREER INVESTIGATION CHECKLIST

Using appropriate information from *Your Career in Healthcare,* research and answer the questions below before you make a final career decision. (You may want to research and answer questions for a second or even a third choice if you are not comfortable with what you learn.)

Career: ....

1. What education and training are required?
   ....
   ....

2. How long will it take to complete the required education and training?
   ....

3. How much money will I need to begin career preparation? ....

   How much money will I need to complete career preparation? ....

4. How will I get all of the career preparation money I need (grants, scholarships, low-cost loans, part-time jobs)?
   ....
   ....
   ....

5. What short-term sacrifices must I make to pursue this career?
   ....
   ....
   ....

6. How will this career decision affect others in my life? What changes and/or sacrifices will they have to make?

   ....
   ....
   ....

7. What characteristics do I have that make this a good career choice for me?

   ....
   ....
   ....

8. Ten years from now, if I am working in my chosen career, I expect my life to be different in the following ways:

   ....
   ....
   ....

Appendix D

INFORMATION INTERVIEW WITH A PROFESSIONAL*

To learn more about an occupation, talk to someone who has done the work you want to do. Introduce yourself, explaining that you need firsthand information about the profession. (Before making a "cold call," ask a relative or friend for names of people in the field. Using the name of a person the professional knows will assure a smoother introduction.)

1. How did you decide to become a ....?

2. What kinds of education and training were required? ....

3. How did you get your first job in the field? ....

4. What do you like best about being a ....?

5. What do you like least about being a ....?

6. How has this kind of work changed since you got into it?
   ....

7. What do you do during a typical day?
   ....

8. What are the most important skills (or knowledge, or attitude) necessary to be a successful ....?

9. Aside from formal training, what kinds of experience should I try to get that would help me prepare to be a ....?

10. What reading would you suggest that would help me learn more about being a
    ....?

11. Who else would you recommend I talk with to find out more about being a
    ....?

Possible additional questions:

....
....
....
....
....
....
....
....

----
* Adapted from *Career Mapper*, produced by Profiles International, Inc., Waco, Texas, © 1995. Distributor: J. L. Krug & Associates, Geneva, IL. With permission.

Index

Academic preparation, 9–10, 14 *See also:* Specific careers
Acute Care Nurse, résumé, sample, 232–233
Aging, 3
Alternative medicine, 7
   veterinary, 148
Anesthetist, nurse, 5, 46–48
Anesthesiologist, 44–46
   assistant, 49–50
Anesthesiology, career opportunities, 44–50
   anesthesiologist, 44–46
      assistant, 49–50
   nurse anesthetist, 5, 46–48
Animal Attendant, 151
Animal Therapists, 122
Anorexia nervosa, 99–100
Audiologist, 114

Binge eating disorder, 99–100
Biomedical Engineer, 96–98
Biomedical Engineering, career opportunities, 90–98
   biomedical engineer, 96–98
   human genetic counselor, 92–93
Blood Bank Technologists, 94
Bulimia nervosa, 99–100

Cardiologist, 52
Cardiology, 20
   management, résumé, sample, 214
   nurse, résumé, sample, 196–197
Cardiovascular:
  diseases, 20
  medicine:
     career opportunities, 51–58
      cardiologist, 52
      cardiovascular technologist, 52–53
      EKG technician, 53–54
         trainee, 153
      perfusionist, 55–56
      respiratory therapist, 57–58
     history, 54–55
     technologist, 52–53
Career assessment, 10–13
Carpal Tunnel Syndrome, 4
Certified Alcohol and Drug Abuse Counselor (CADAC), 106–107
Certified Registered Nurse Anesthetists (CRNA), 5
   résumé, sample, 215
Charting, computerized, 36
Clinical Chemistry Technologists, 94
Coding Specialist, 87–88
Compensation, negotiating, 282–283
Computerized charting, 36
Confidentiality, patient records, 87
Cost containment, 5
Counselor:
   grief, résumé, sample, 254–255
   professional, 107–109
   résumé, sample, 248–249
Cover letters, 171–175
Curriculum Vitae, 170 *See also:* Résumés
Cytotechnologists, 94

Database services, 260
Dental:
   assistant, 151
   hygienist, 66–67
   laboratory technician, 68–69
Dentist, 59–63
Dentistry:
   career opportunities, 59–69
     dental:
       assistant, 151
       hygienist, 66–67
       laboratory technician, 68–69
     dentist, 59–63

endodontist, 63
   oral maxillofacial surgeon, 63
   oral pathologist, 65
   orthodontist, 65
   pediatric dentist, 65
   periodontist, 65
   prosthodontist, 65–66
   public health dentist, 66
  history, 66
Dermatologist, 21
Diagnostic Instrumentation Executive,
   résumé, sample, 222–224
Diagnostic Medical Sonographer, 141–142
Dialysis Technician, 152
Dietetic Technician, 74–75
Dietetics, career opportunities, 70–75
   dietetic technician, 74–75
   dietitian, 70–74
     résumé, sample, 206–207, 250–251
Dietitian, 70–74
   résumé, sample, 206–207, 250–251
Dispensing Optician Trainee, 152
Doctors, career opportunities, 15–29
Down's Syndrome, 92–93

Eating disorders, 99–100
Educational requirements, 9–10, 14 See
   also: Specific career
EKG:
   technician, 53–54
     trainee, 153
   technologist trainee, 152–153
Emergency Medical Technician, 153–154
Emergency Medicine, 20, 27
Employment:
   agencies, 256–257
   trends, 257–258
Endodontist, 63
Environmental Health Officer, 130
Epidemiologist, 130
Ether, first use of, 59–60
Ethnopharmacy, 116
Executive recruiters, 257–258

Eyecare, career opportunities, 76–82
   dispensing optician trainee, 152
   ophthalmic:
     laboratory technician, 81–82
     medical technician/technologist, 78–79
   ophthalmologist, 76
   optician, 80–81
   optometrist, 77–78

Family Physician, 21–22
   résumé, sample, 183–184
Family Practice, 20, 27

Gardening as therapy, 126
Grief Counselor, résumé, sample, 254–255
Growth of the healthcare profession, 2–5
Gynecologist, 24
   résumé, sample, 188–189
Gynecology, 20, 27

Health Maintenance Organizations, 5–6
Healthcare:
   areas of study, 6–7
   professions:
     growth, 2–5
     volatility, 5–6
Heart disease, 51
Health Educator, 130
Health Information Management, career
     opportunities, 83–89
   coding specialist, 87–88
   medical record:
     administrator, 84–85
     technician, 85–86
   medical transcriptionist, 88–89
High School Graduates, career opportuni-
     ties, 150–157
   animal attendant, 151
   dental assistant, 151
   dialysis technician, 152
   dispensing optician trainee, 152
   EEG technologist trainee, 152–153
   EKG technician trainee, 153

emergency medical technician, 153–154
home health aide, 154
medical assistant, 156
nursing aide, 156–157
psychiatric aide, 156–157
Histology Technician, 95
Home Health Aide, 154
Home test kits, 96
Hospice Movement, 104
administrator, résumé, sample, 225–226
Human Genetic Counselor, 92–93

Immunology Technologists, 94
Internal Medicine, 20, 27
Internist, 24
Interview:
first, 274–279
first impression, 274–275
preparation, 271–273
second, 281–282
techniques, 269–283
thank you letter, 279–280

Laboratory Medicine, career opportunities, 90–98
blood bank technologists, 94
clinical chemistry technologists, 94
cytotechnologists, 94
dialysis technician, 152
EEG technologist trainee, 152–153
EKG technician trainee, 153
histology technician, 95
human genetic counselor, 92–93
immunology technologists, 94
medical technician, 95
medical technologist, 93–95
microbiology technologists, 94
pathologist, 90–91
assistant, 91–92
phlebotomist, 95
Laboratory Technician, résumé, sample, 217, 238
Licensed Practical Nurse, 38

Managed Care Marketing Executive, résumé, sample, 227–228
Maxillofacial Surgeon, résumé, sample, 185–187
Medical:
assistant, 156
résumé, sample, 241
doctors (M.D.), 16 *See also:* Physicians' specialties, 20
instrumentation management, résumé, sample, 239–240
record:
administrator, 84–85
technician, 85–86
sales and marketing, résumé, sample, 243–244
school, 17
technician, 95
technologist, 93–95
résumé, sample, 242
transcriptionist, 88–89
Mental Health:
career opportunities, 99–109
certified alcohol and drug abuse counselor (CADAC), 106–107
mental health social worker, 105–106
outreach worker, 107
professional counselor, 107–109
psychiatric:
aide, 156–157
technician, 101–102
psychiatrist, 100–101
psychologist, 103–104
social worker, 105–106
Microbiology Technologists, 94
Midwife, nurse, 36–37

Natural medicine, 7
Networking, 261
online, 263–268
Neurologist, 24
Newspaper advertisements, 258–260, 269
blind ads, 260

Index

Nuclear Medicine Technologist, 142–143
Nurse:
  acute care, résumé, sample, 232–233
  anesthetist, 46–48
  executive, 41–42
    résumé, sample, 229–230
  licensed practical, 38
  manager, 41
    résumé, sample, 199–202
  midwife, 36–37
  practitioner, 34–35
  résumé, sample, 196–204
Nursing Aide, 156–157
Nursing, career opportunities, 30–42
  home health aide, 154
  licensed practical nurse, 38
  medical assistant, 156
  nurse:
    executive, 41–42
    midwife, 36–37
    practitioner, 34–35
  nursing aide, 156–157
  registered nurses (RN), 30–34

Obstetrician, 24
Obstetrics, 20, 27
  résumé, sample, 188–189
Occupational:
  health nurse, 130
  therapist, 125–126
    résumé, sample, 245
  therapy:
    assistant, 127
    career opportunities, 120–128
      occupational therapist, 125–126
      occupational therapy assistant, 127
Ophthalmic:
  laboratory technician, 81–82
  medical technician/technologist, 78–79
Ophthalmologist, 76
Optician, 80–81
Optometrist, 77–78
  résumé, sample, 208–209

Oral:
  maxillofacial surgeon, 63
  pathologist, 65
Orthodontist, 65
Orthopedic Surgery, 20
Osteopathic Doctors (D.O.), 16–19
  résumé, sample, 190–192
  specialties, 20
Otolaryngologist, 24
Outreach Worker, 107

Pathologist, 24–25, 27, 90–91
  assistant, 91–92
Pediatric Dentist, 65
Pediatrician, 25
Pediatrics, 20, 27
Perfusionist, 55–56
Periodontist, 65
Personal Fitness Trainer, résumé, sample, 236–237
Pharmacist, 115–117
  assistant, 118
  résumé, sample, 210
Pharmacy, career opportunities, 115–119
  pharmacist, 115–117
    assistant, 118
Phlebotomist, 95
Physiatrist, 25
Physical Therapist, 120–122
  assistant, 124
  résumé, sample, 218–219
Physical Therapy, career opportunities, 120–128
  physical therapist, 120–122
    assistant, 124
Physicians, 16–20
  assistant, 27–29, 246–247
  earnings, 27
  educational preparation, 17
  outlook, 26
  personality qualities, 16
  prerequisites, 16
  principal duties, 19

Index

résumé, sample, 178–194
specialties, 20–22
temporary services, 263
Podiatrist, 25
Positive suggestions, power of, 46
Proctologist, 26
Professional Counselor, 107–109
Prosthodontist, 65–66
Psychiatric:
   aide, 156–157
   technician, 101–102
Psychiatrist, 100–101
Psychiatry, 20, 27
Psychologist, 103–104
   résumé, sample, 248–249
Public health, 3–4
   career opportunities, 128–135
      environmental health officer, 130
      epidemiologist, 130
      health educator, 130
      occupational health nurse, 130
      public health:
         dentist, 66
         nurse, résumé, sample, 203–204
         statistician, 130
   history, 129

Radiation Therapist, 138–139
Radiographer, 140–141
Radiologist, 136–138
   résumé, sample, 178–182
Radiology, 20, 27
   career opportunities, 136–143
      diagnostic medical sonographer, 141–142
      nuclear medicine technologist, 142–143
      radiation therapist, 138–139
      radiographer, 140–141
      radiologist, 136–138
   director of, résumé, sample, 216
   history of, 139–140

Registered Nurses (RN), 30–34
   résumé, sample, 198, 235
Respiratory Therapist, 57–58
   résumé, sample, 252
Résumé development, 160–170
   components, 164–166
   experience, 168
   formats, 162–163
   Internet, using, 170
   organization, 161–162
   targeting, 163–164

Sign language, 114
Social Worker, résumé, sample, 234
Speech-Language Pathologist, 110–113
   résumé, sample, 211–212, 253
Speech-Language Pathology, career opportunities, 110–114
   audiologist, 114
   speech-language pathologist, 110–113
Standard Occupational Classification codes, 296–297
Surgery, 20, 27

Trade publications, 260

Urologist, 26

Veterinarian, 144–145
   résumé, sample, 193–194
Veterinary Medicine, career opportunities, 144–149
   animal attendant, 151
   veterinary technician, 148–149
Vision:
   brain injury, 78
   headaches, 79–80

X Chromosome, 92–93
X-Ray technician, résumé, sample, 220

Yoga, 7–8

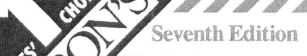

Students' #1 Choice

BARRON'S

Seventh Edition

MCAT

How to Prepare for the Medical College Admission Test

Hugo R. Seibel, Ph.D., Kenneth E. Guyer, Ph.D.,
Anthony B. Mangum, Ph.D., C. M. Conway, Ph.D.,
Arthur F. Conway, Ph.D. and Wesley L. Shanholtzer, Ph.D.

Updated to Reflect the All-New Exam Format

Deals with the newly defined subject areas and redesigned question types —exactly as you'll find them on the new MCAT

Four Complete and Updated Practice Tests all in the New Format

Complete with Answers and Explanations to All Questions

Revised and Updated Subject Review Sections

Science and Math Reviews • Strategies for the new Verbal Reasoning exam • How to Write the Essay

Barron's Educational Series, Inc. $12.95 Canada $16.95

$12.95   Canada $16.95   **ISBN: 0-8120-4646-3**

Books may be purchased at your bookstore, or by mail from Barron's. Enclose check or money order for the total amount plus sales tax where applicable and 10% for postage and handling charge (minimum charge $3.75, Canada $4.00). Prices subject to change without notice.

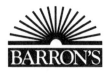

Barron's Educational Series, Inc.
250 Wireless Boulevard • Hauppauge, New York 11788
In Canada: Georgetown Book Warehouse
34 Armstrong Avenue • Georgetown, Ontario L7G 4R9

(#42) 4/96

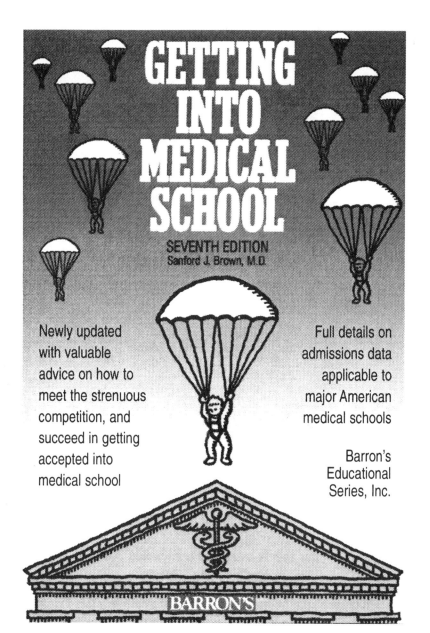

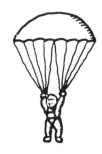

"Majoring in non-science will probably raise your overall GPA and put you in a more advantageous position when seeking admission..."

"Apart from their annual pilgrimage to a medical school (a trip which you can more profitably make on your own), the value of [premedical clubs] is dubious..."

"The premedical advisor holds no degree or certification for the job, is not licensed, and is not subject to peer review. The adviser is only as good as personal interest and involvement allow."

The hardest obstacle to overcome in becoming a physician is getting admitted to a medical school. This book cuts through the official jargon and tells you exactly what you really need to do to be accepted. How to choose a college and a major field of study, how to avoid the "Premed Syndrome," how to cope with the MCAT, when, where, and how to apply to medical school, and how to deal with rejections. With a directory of AMA-approved medical schools.

$10.95 Canada $14.50

Barron's Educational Series, Inc.
250 Wireless Boulevard, Hauppauge, New York 11788
In Canada: Georgetown Book Warehouse
34 Armstrong Avenue, Georgetown, Ontario L7G 4R9
Please send me the following quantities:

_____GETTING INTO MEDICAL SCHOOL $10.95, Can. $14.50
ISBN: 0-8120-4266-2
I am enclosing a check for_____which includes applicable sales tax plus 10% transportation charges (minimum charge $3.75, Can. $4.00). Price subject to change without notice.

Name _____

Address _____

City_____ State _____ Zip _____

(#37) 7/96